Fetal Medicine and Genetics

Fetal Medicine and Genetics

Editors

Sumitra Bachani

MD MNAMS Fellow Maternal Fetal Medicine (AIIMS, New Delhi)
Expert in Fetal Medicine (BC Natal FMRC Barcelona)
Professor, Senior Specialist, and Lead Faculty
Fetal Medicine & Genetic Clinic
Department of Obstetrics and Gynecology
Vardhman Mahavir Medical College and Safdarjung Hospital
New Delhi, India

Manisha Kumar

MBBS MS FICOG Expert in Fetal Medicine (BC Natal FMRC Barcelona)
Director-Professor
Department of Obstetrics and Gynecology
In charge of Fetal Medicine
Lady Hardinge Medical College
New Delhi, India

Forewords

Ashok Khurana

Pratima Mittal

JAYPEE

JAYPEE BROTHERS MEDICAL PUBLISHERS

The Health Sciences Publisher

New Delhi | London

JAYPEE **Jaypee Brothers Medical Publishers (P) Ltd**

Headquarters
Jaypee Brothers Medical Publishers (P) Ltd
EMCA House, 23/23-B
Ansari Road, Daryaganj
New Delhi 110 002, India
Landline: +91-11-23272143, +91-11-23272703
+91-11-23282021, +91-11-23245672
Email: jaypee@jaypeebrothers.com

Corporate Office
Jaypee Brothers Medical Publishers (P) Ltd
4838/24, Ansari Road, Daryaganj
New Delhi 110 002, India
Phone: +91-11-43574357
Fax: +91-11-43574314
Email: jaypee@jaypeebrothers.com

Overseas Office
JP Medical Ltd.
83, Victoria Street, London
SW1H 0HW (UK)
Phone: +44 20 3170 8910
Fax: +44 (0)20 3008 6180
Email: info@jpmedpub.com

Website: www.jaypeebrothers.com
Website: www.jaypeedigital.com

Inquiries for bulk sales may be solicited at: jaypee@jaypeebrothers.com

Fetal Medicine and Genetics

First Edition: **2024**

ISBN: 978-93-5696-846-2

Printed in India at Sterling Graphics Pvt. Ltd.

Dedicated to

Arunav, Mansi and Javin our first students and critics

Contributors

Akshatha Prabhu
Fellowship in Fetal Medicine (FMF UK) MRCOG (UK) MS (Obs and Gyne)
Senior Consultant
Department of Fetal Medicine
Indraprastha Apollo Hospitals
New Delhi, India

Alok Varshney MD DNB (Radiology)
Senior Consultant Radiologist
Department of Radiology
Central Diagnostics
New Delhi, India

Ankita Jain
MBBS DNB (Obs and Gyne) ICOG Fellow (Critical Care Obstetrics)
Assistant Professor
Department of Obstetrics and Gynecology
Vardhman Mahavir Medical College and Safdarjung Hospital
New Delhi, India

Aprajita Gupta MD (Obs and Gyne)
Fellow National Board Maternal Fetal Medicine
Department of Obstetrics and Gynecology
Vardhman Mahavir Medical College and Safdarjung Hospital, New Delhi, India

Bijoya Mukherjee
MS (Obs and Gyne) DNB (Obs and Gyne) Fellowship in Fetal Medicine
Fellow
Department of Fetal Medicine
Indraprastha Apollo Hospitals
Kolkata, West Bengal, India

Chanchal Singh MD (Obs and Gyne) MRCOG FICOG
Lead Consultant
Department of Fetal Medicine, Obstetrics and Gynecology
Madhukar Rainbow Children's Hospital and BirthRight, by Rainbow Hospitals
New Delhi, India

Harshiba Kaur MD (Obs and Gyne) DNB MRCOG
Associate Consultant
Department of Fetal Medicine, Obstetrics and Gynecology
Madhukar Rainbow Children's Hospital and BirthRight, by Rainbow Hospitals
New Delhi, India

Jaya Chawla
MS FICMCH Fellow Maternal Fetal Medicine (AIIMS)
Professor
Department of Obstetrics and Gynecology
Atal Bihari Vajpayee Institute of Medical Sciences and Dr Ram Manohar Lohia Hospital
New Delhi, India

Jyotsna Suri MBBS MD FICOG
Professor and Consultant
Department of Obstetrics and Gynecology
Vardhman Mahavir Medical College and Safdarjung Hospital
New Delhi, India

K Aparna Sharma
MD DNB MICOG MNAMS MFM Fellow
Professor
Department of Obstetrics and Gynecology
All India Institute of Medical Sciences
New Delhi, India

K Manikandan MD DNB MRCOG PDF-FM
Lead Consultant in Fetal Therapy
Department of Fetal Medicine
The Fetal Clinic
Ellaipillaichavady, Puducherry, India

Manisha Kumar
MBBS MS FICOG Expert in Fetal Medicine (BC Natal FMRC Barcelona)
Director-Professor
Department of Obstetrics and Gynecology
In charge of Fetal Medicine
Lady Hardinge Medical College
New Delhi, India

Meena Lall PhD (Human Genetics-Applied Biology)
Senior Consultant and Professor
Department of Genetics
Institute of Medical Genetics and Genomics
Sir Ganga Ram Hospital
New Delhi, India

Mounika Endrakanti MD DM
Consultant (Research)
Department of Pediatrics
All India Institute of Medical Sciences
New Delhi, India

Neerja Gupta MD DM
Additional Professor
Department of Pediatrics
All India Institute of Medical Sciences
New Delhi, India

Nikhil Kapoor DMRD
Consultant Radiologist
Sattva the Fetal Medicine Centre
New Delhi, India

Noopur Chawla Pruthi
MBBS DNB (Obs and Gyne)
Fellow National Board Maternal Fetal Medicine
Department of Obstetrics and Gynecology
Vardhman Mahavir Medical College and
Safdarjung Hospital, New Delhi, India

Poonam Tara
MBBS MD (Obs and Gyne) FRCOG (London) Diploma in Advanced Obstetric Scan (UK)
Senior Consultant
Department of Obstetrics
Gynecology and Fetal Medicine
Centre for Fetal Maternal Care
New Delhi, India

Poornima Sharma MD (Obs and Gyne)
Fellow National Board Maternal Fetal Medicine
Department of Obstetrics and Gynecology
Vardhman Mahavir Medical College and
Safdarjung Hospital, New Delhi, India

Preeti Paliwal PhD
Senior Scientist and Associate Professor
Department of Genetics
Institute of Medical Genetics and Genomics
Sir Ganga Ram Hospital
New Delhi, India

Ratna Dua Puri MD DM (Medical Genetics)
Head
Department of Genetics
Institute of Medical Genetics and Genomics
Sir Ganga Ram Hospital
New Delhi, India

Reema Bhatt MS DNB FICOG MNAMS
Professor and Head
Department of Fetal Medicine and Perinatology
Amrita Institute and Research Centre
Faridabad, Haryana, India

Reena Yadav DGO MD FICOG
Director Professor and Head
Department of Obstetrics and Gynecology
Lady Hardinge Medical College and
Smt Sucheta Kriplani Hospital
New Delhi, India

Rinshi Abid Elayedatt
MS DGO DNB Fellowship in Maternal-Fetal Medicine
Diploma of Expert in Imaging in MFM
Clinical Assistant Professor
Department of Fetal Medicine and Perinatology
Amrita Institute
Kochi, Kerala, India

Ritika Bajaj
MBBS MS (Obs and Gyne) Fellowship in MFM (AIIMS, New Delhi)
Consultant Fetal Medicine
Department of Maternal Fetal Medicine,
Obstetrics and Gynecology
Jindal IVF and Sant Memorial Hospital
Chandigarh, India

Saloni Kamboj MBBS MS DNB
Scientist C
Department of Obstetrics and Gynecology
All India Institute of Medical Sciences
New Delhi, India

Sangeeta Gupta MD FRCOG
Director-Professor
Department of Obstetrics and Gynecology
Maulana Azad Medical College
New Delhi, India

Seema Thakur
MBBS MS (Obs and Gyne) DM (Medical Genetics)
Senior Consultant
Department of Genetic and Fetal Diagnosis
Fortis Hospital and Rainbow Children Hospital
New Delhi, India

Shilpa Thakur CGC
Genetic Counselor
Sattva the Fetal Medicine Centre
New Delhi, India

Shreya Singh Kushwaha MD (Obs and Gyne)
Fellow National Board Maternal Fetal Medicine
Department of Obstetrics and Gynecology
Vardhman Mahavir Medical College and
Safdarjung Hospital, New Delhi, India

Suchandana Dasgupta MBBS MS FNB (MFM)
Senior Resident
Department of Obstetrics and Gynecology
Vardhman Mahavir Medical College and
Safdarjung Hospital
New Delhi, India

Sudha Kohli PhD
Consultant
Department of Molecular Genetics
Institute of Medical Genetics and Genomics
Sir Ganga Ram Hospital
New Delhi, India

Sudhisha Dubey Mphil PhD
Senior Consultant
Department of Genetics
Institute of Medical Genetics and Genomics
Sir Ganga Ram Hospital
New Delhi, India

Sumitra Bachani
MD MNAMS Fellow Maternal Fetal Medicine (AIIMS, New Delhi) Expert in Fetal Medicine (BC Natal FMRC Barcelona)
Professor, Senior Specialist, and Lead Faculty
Fetal Medicine & Genetic Clinic
Department of Obstetrics and Gynecology
Vardhman Mahavir Medical College and
Safdarjung Hospital
New Delhi, India

Sunil Jaiman MBBS MD Dip RCPath (UK)
Pathology Discipline Director and Human
Disease Foundation-I Course Director,
Assistant Professor
Department of Pathology
Wayne State University School of Medicine
Detroit, MI, USA

Vandana Chaddha
MS (Obs and Gyne) Clinical Fellow Maternal-Fetal Medicine University of Toronto
Consultant
Department of Fetal Medicine
Sattva the Fetal Medicine Centre
New Delhi, India

Veronica Arora MBBS MD DM (Medical Genetics)
Consultant
Department of Genetics
Institute of Medical Genetics and Genomics
Sir Ganga Ram Hospital
New Delhi, India

Vivek Krishnan
MS DGO DNB Fellowship in Fetal Medicine
Clinical Associate Professor and Head
Department of Fetal Medicine and Perinatology
Amrita Institute
Kochi, Kerala, India

Foreword

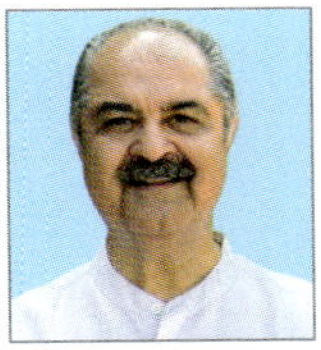

Dear Readers,

When Dr Sumitra Bachani and Dr Manisha Kumar told me that they were putting together a textbook of fetal medicine and related genetics especially curated for postgraduates and clinicians, I was truly pleased. Not for one reason but two. The first reason was that this is truly the need of the hour. A rapidly advancing field today, interdisciplinary updated content, and awareness of fetal medicine need to be presented in a way that is simple yet exhaustive. We need a single book that brings together current imaging technology, progress in genetics, and high-risk obstetrics and perinatology, in the perspective of obstetric, neonatal, and pediatric specialty practice. The chapters of this book do substantial justice to this endeavor. The second reason that brought me pleasure is that the quality of the book is a foregone conclusion. I say this because I know the editors and authors well. In their dual role of clinician and teacher, they steer their professional paths with excellence. I greatly appreciate the way they conduct practice and teaching of the subject: Sumitra Bachani at Vardhman Mahavir Medical College and Safdarjung Hospital and Manisha Kumar at Sucheta Kriplani Hospital associated with Lady Hardinge Medical College. The efficient and practical fetal medicine units that they have set up in these teaching hospitals of New Delhi reflect continuing hours of dedication, sacrifice, and devotion that they put in. Their rapid translation of research findings into clinical practice in spite of resource restrictions is truly admirable.

The book guides you through applied basics, pathophysiology, daily practice, guidelines, protocols, checklists, and problem solving in a remarkably comfortable and exemplary way. The chapters take you through elements of screening, fetal ultrasound, genetics, fetal growth, and a host of subject headings in a systematic and easily doable way. Authors of chapters are all experts in their field.

It is a must-have book for postgraduates students in obstetrics and gynecology, radiology, and genetics as well as for practitioners who wish to update their practice. The "Quiz" in between the chapters is the icing on the cake and offers rapid revision.

In essence, the highlight of the book is that it presents easy-to-achieve excellence for the novice.

I highly recommend this book for all professionals in fetal health care.

Ashok Khurana MD
Professor
Mentor Emeritus
Society of Fetal Medicine
Chairman and Consultant in Reproductive Ultrasound
The Ultrasound Lab
New Delhi, India

Foreword

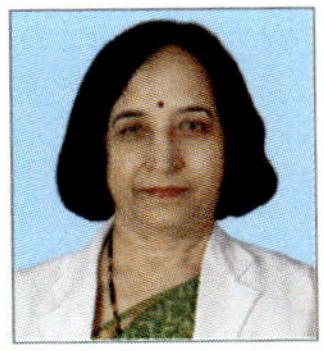

As the field of obstetrics and gynecology is now expanding into subspecialties, in today's dynamic medical landscape, the field of obstetrics and fetal medicine stands at the forefront of innovation and compassion. It is a discipline where science intertwines with the miracle of life, where meticulous care meets profound joy, and where every milestone is a testament to the resilience of the human spirit. The field is evolving every day and I am sure this book will fulfill the requirements of fellows, postgraduate students, obstetricians and practitioners of fetal medicine as knowledge of this field is necessary to complete the modern obstetric care which now focuses on both the mother and fetus dyad.

It is a pleasure to write about the book editors Sumitra Bachani and Manisha Kumar. I have known both of them at different times during my tenure as Head of Unit and Head of Department of Obstetrics and Gynecology at Vardhman Mahavir Medical College and Safdarjung Hospital, New Delhi, India. As is my desire to see my juniors grow in ability and skills, Dr Sumitra Bachani completed her Fellowship in Maternal Fetal Medicine from All India Institute of Medical Sciences, New Delhi while I was heading the department and subsequently she worked toward expanding the special clinic of Fetal Medicine to incorporate fetal invasive procedures and fetal therapy such as intrauterine transfusion and radiofrequency ablation at Safdarjung Hospital. She has a keen interest in teaching and is passionate about her work in fetal medicine.

Dr Manisha Kumar has worked in Safdarjung Hospital at the beginning of her career as Senior Resident. She was hard working and diligent. After completing her tenure, she went on to do 2 years senior residency in Medical Genetics from Sanjay Gandhi Postgraduate Institute of Medical Sciences (SGPGI), Lucknow, Uttar Pradesh. She has established fetal medicine facility and genetic lab at Lady Hardinge Medical College, New Delhi. She has been actively involved in research in the fields of preeclampsia, stillbirth, and birth defects. She was part of the World Health Organization (WHO) project "Stillbirth and Birth Defect" registry in seven hospitals of Delhi, where I was the Principal Investigator. She has numerous publications in this field, mostly in international journals, providing a good account of the outcome of various birth defects in our part of the world.

It was my final injunction to Dr Sumitra to start thinking of a book on fetal medicine for postgraduates as this was a lacuna in their teaching. I am really happy to know that she has taken positive steps toward it and brought it to fruition. The chapters cover the most needed topics in fetal medicine and genetics. The authors are the best faculty and well-known teachers in their field.

I wish both of them all the success in achieving their desire of bringing fetal medicine within the grasp of postgraduates, general obstetricians and fetal medicine specialists.

With warmest regards,

Pratima Mittal
Professor, Senior Consultant, and Head
Department of Obstetrics and Gynecology
Amrita Institute of Medical Sciences and Research Center
Faridabad, Haryana, India

Preface

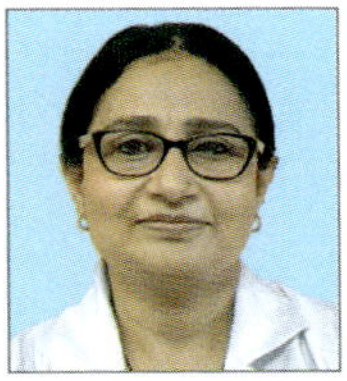

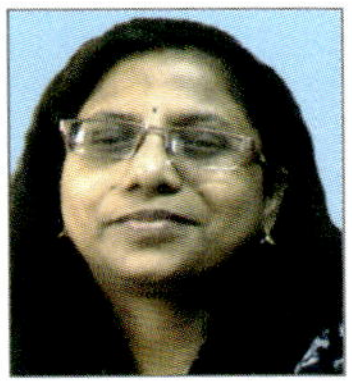

Sumitra Bachani **Manisha Kumar**

We are grateful that you picked up this book! It was a spontaneous conception, a bit of an arduous progression but a smooth delivery. It is a unique amalgamation of basics and some advanced topics relatable to both postgraduates, general obstetricians and fellows in maternal fetal medicine who can keep it as reference for working knowledge. The postgraduates will find it very convenient as all the basic topics in fetal medicine such as preconception counseling to prenatal tests and fetal therapy are provided in a compact form. The students can challenge themselves by first attempting the quiz and then read up the chapter related to it.

The authors of each chapter have tailored the writeup such that it is easily grasped and benefits the residents and general obstetricians. It is up-to-date with ready references for further reading. The book is just the beginning of our effort to bring together relevant topics of fetal medicine. We look forward to adding more topics in future editions. We hope you will enjoy reading the book as much as we did while putting it together. We look forward to your constructive feedback to make this even more better.

Acknowledgments

We would like to thank our family, especially Dr Kamal Bachani and Dr Rajesh Kumar, friends and colleagues for supporting us all through our journey.

Our special thanks to each other for working together from conceptualizing to the printing of this book.

We are filled with gratitude towards our authors, who are the pioneers in their field and have given their best in spite of their busy schedule.

We are grateful to our publishers M/s Jaypee Brothers Medical Publishers (P) Ltd, New Delhi, India, for working tirelessly to make our dream of bringing out this book a reality.

We would like to acknowledge that we have always considered ourselves fortunate to be teachers, and have learnt a lot from our students. We would send our deepest prayers to each of our patients, who have trusted us and have shown exemplary courage in their tough times. The acknowledgment cannot be complete without our gratitude towards our teachers, who have played a major role in making us who we are today.

Lastly, we would be ever indebted to our parents, our philosopher guide and Almighty for giving us this valuable life and guiding us to create value.

Contents

CHAPTER 1

Preconceptional Care and Teratogenesis

Jyotsna Suri, Ankita Jain

KEY POINTS

1. Preconceptional care is a part of preventive care that includes screening for pregnancy related risk factors *before pregnancy,* educating the couple about those risks and the management options; and intervention for optimization of the woman's condition to provide for optimum pregnancy outcome.
2. A structured form or checklist aids in obtaining a thorough history and identifying the risk factors.
3. Chronic medical ailments should be optimized before embarking on a pregnancy.
4. Women with high-risk history should undergo genetic counseling.
5. Core preconception interventions that can reduce the occurrence of congenital disorders, fetal growth abnormalities, and pregnancy complications include folic acid supplementation and intake of fortified foods, glycemic control in women with diabetes, abstinence from alcohol and illicit drugs and smoking cessation, reduction of obesity, avoidance of teratogens, vaccinations, and behavioral changes to reduce the risk of acquiring infections such as toxoplasmosis, cytomegalovirus, and sexually transmitted infections (STIs).
6. A teratogen is an agent that acts during embryonic or fetal development to produce a permanent alteration of form and function causing structural abnormalities. It can result in fetal death, fetal growth restriction, birth defects, and impaired neurological development.
7. The teratogenic effect is dependent on various factors such as duration and timing of exposure, dose and peak effect of teratogen, gender, and genetic predisposition.
8. A teratogenic exposure during critical periods of organogenesis can result in major structural defects. Hence, exposure to these agents must be avoided during these critical periods of organ development.

INTRODUCTION

Preconception care refers to the process of identifying social, behavioral, environmental, and biomedical risks to a woman's fertility and pregnancy outcome and then reducing these risks through education, counseling, and appropriate intervention before conception.[1] Preconception intervention is more important than antenatal intervention for the prevention of congenital anomalies since as many as 30% of pregnant women begin traditional prenatal care in the second trimester (>13 weeks of gestation), which is after the primary period of organogenesis. Preconception care should be an essential part of primary and preventive care.[2,3]

The three integral components of preconception care are:

1. *Screening:* This involves identification of risk factors related to pregnancy.
2. *Imparting information and counseling:* Patient education regarding pregnancy risks, management options, and reproductive alternatives.
3. *Interventions:* Initiation of interventions, when possible, to provide optimum pregnancy outcome.

TARGET POPULATION

The target population for preconception care is any woman in the reproductive age group who desires childbearing in the future and should not be restricted to women who are planning pregnancy imminently. The women who seek gynecological consult for any indication, family planning services, after a negative pregnancy test, and those visiting the postpartum clinic are some of the women who should receive preconception counseling. Besides women coming to a general practitioner or physician for nongynecological reasons would also benefit from this; hence, it is imperative that all physicians and healthcare providers along with the obstetrician and gynecologist should be sensitized in their undergraduate training about this very crucial aspect of primary care.

Addressing the preconceptional issues with the women in the reproductive age group at any point of their contact with the healthcare system is desirable because more than half the pregnancies are unplanned. Furthermore, in our country, there are very few dedicated preconceptional counseling centers.

Factors which facilitate the process of counseling are preconceptional care checklists, patient information sheets in local and simple language, posters and video films in the patient-waiting areas, and availability of dedicated healthcare providers.

COMPONENTS OF PRECONCEPTIONAL HEALTH PACKAGE[4]

Screening

- Screening of the couple through a detailed medical and family history, including genetic history of the patient, spouse, and family **(Box 1)**, followed by examination
- Screening to identify ABO and Rh(D) blood type to detect possibility of blood incompatibility between would-be couple
- Hemoglobin levels to identify anemia
- Screening to detect hemoglobinopathies, e.g., sickle cell anemia and thalassemia if suspected by family history, examination and red cell indices
- Screening to detect infectious diseases such as human immunodeficiency virus (HIV), hepatitis B and C, and syphilis as suggested by history and examination
- Screening to detect sexually transmitted diseases [other than syphilis, HIV, and Hepatitis B virus (HBV)] such as gonorrhea and chlamydia as indicated by history
- Screening for diabetes, hypertension, a thyroid disorders and organ dysfunction such as liver and kidney. If directed by family history or examination
- Screening for obesity/underweight
- Identifying rubella immunity of women
- Psychosocial and domestic issues should be identified and women with mental health issues should be referred to a psychiatrist.

Information and Counseling

- *Timing of pregnancy:* The optimum biological age for pregnancy is between

BOX 1: Genetic history of patient, spouse, and family.[10]

- *History of congenital abnormalities:*
  - Neural tube defects
  - Heart defects
  - Cleft lip/palate
  - Any other
- *Chromosomal abnormalities:*
  - Down syndrome
  - Mental retardation/learning disabilities (fragile X syndrome)
- Advanced maternal or paternal age
- *Inherited diseases:*
  - Hemoglobinopathy
  - Muscular dystrophy
  - Thrombophilia
  - Cystic fibrosis
  - Huntington's chorea
  - Hemophilia
  - Metabolic disorders (e.g., phenylketonuria, diabetes)
  - Kidney disease
  - Deafness
  - Marfan syndrome
  - Any other
- *Ethnicity:*
  - Eastern European (Ashkenazi) Jews (Tay–Sachs, Canavan risk, etc.)
  - French Canadian or Cajun (Tay–Sachs risk)
  - Mediterranean region (hemoglobinopathy risk)
  - Asia, including Southeast Asia and Western Pacific (hemoglobinopathy risk)
  - Africa and Middle East (hemoglobinopathy risk)
  - South America and Caribbean (hemoglobinopathy risk)
  - Caucasian (cystic fibrosis)
- Consanguinity
- Recurrent pregnancy loss, stillbirth, or early infant death
- Maternal metabolic disorder

20 and 35 years of age. Pregnancy at an earlier or later age entails additional morbidities for both the mother and the child. There is three times increased risk of hypertension in women with advanced maternal age, besides the risk of placenta previa, gestational diabetes, preterm birth, and increased cesarean section rate.[5] There is also an increased risk of poor perinatal outcomes, in terms of increased still births, perinatal mortality, low birth weight, and nursery admissions. Women should be counseled that advanced maternal age is also associated with an increased risk of conditions such as infertility, fetal aneuploidy miscarriage, and the risk of fetal chromosomal anomalies, in particular Down syndrome, which increases sharply with increasing maternal age.

- Creating awareness about reproductive biology and physiology of pregnancy
- Information about different contraceptive options available for the couple
- Counseling regarding safe sexual practices and sexual behavior
- Counseling regarding ill effects of substance abuse and alcohol
- Counseling about optimizing prepregnancy weight
- Counseling about healthy lifestyle, nutritive diet, and regular exercise
- Information about effect of chronic diseases, genetic disorders, and teratogenic drugs on future childbearing if relevant to the patient.
- *Genetic counseling:* It is the process by which patients at risk of a genetic disorder (identified by taking the genetic history as given in **Box 1**) are informed about the consequences of the disorder, the probability of developing and transmitting it, and the means by which this risk can be reduced. It aims at empowering the couple to take the appropriate decision and course of action in view of the risk. The risk is assessed by taking detailed structured history of previous pregnancy outcomes, chromosomal

disorders, genetic diseases in family, and consanguinity. Consanguineous couples are counseled regarding increased risk of autosomal recessive disorders. A three-generation pedigree chart is made in the cases with suggestive history. The genetic counseling allows couples planning pregnancy to make informed reproductive decisions about adoption, surrogacy, use of donor sperm, in vitro fertilization after preimplantation genetic diagnosis, avoidance of pregnancy, and prenatal diagnosis.

Interventions

- Confirmatory tests if any of the screening test is positive.
- Live vaccines (varicella, measle, mumps, and rubella) should be administered at least 1 month prior to pregnancy.
- Vaccination of eligible partners for hepatitis B. Individuals, whose partner is hepatitis B surface antigen (HBsAg) positive, are given a booster dose of HBV if they have been vaccinated before and a full vaccination course if they have not been vaccinated before.
- Couples with a family history of hemoglobinopathy or any other genetic disease are referred to genetic specialist in the region for further evaluation.
- Referral of persons with chronic disorders to respective specialists so as to ensure good control of disease prior to marriage and pregnancy.
- Administer *folic acid* (400–500 µg daily) supplementation at least 1 month before pregnancy and for 3 months thereafter.[6]
- Women at moderate risk of having babies with neural tube defects (NTD) (family history of NTD and diabetes mellitus) are advised 1 mg folic acid, whereas all women at high risk for NTD [previous history of NTD in woman/partner/previous pregnancy, hemoglobinopathies, body mass index (BMI) >30 kg/m^2, known mutation to MTHFR or on medications affecting folate metabolism, e.g., anti-convulsants] are advised 4 mg folic acid in the periconception period.[6]
- Iron (60 mg weekly) and folic acid (500 µg weekly) supplementation for all women of reproductive age group (20–49 years) under Anemia Mukt Bharat Programme.[7]
- Deworming (Tablet Albendazole 400 mg single dose biannually) for all women of reproductive age group (20–49 years) under Anemia Mukt Bharat Programme.[7]
- Treatment of STIs detected during screening.
- Cessation of smoking, alcohol, and drugs before pregnancy.
- Limit caffeine intake (<200–300 mg daily).
- Only cooked fish should be consumed and fish high in mercury content should be avoided.
- Avoid multivitamin preparations with >5,000 IU of vitamin A (increased risk of teratogenesis at >10,000 IU/day).
- Glycemic control in women with diabetes—the American Diabetes Association (ADA) recommends for a pre-conceptional glycosylated hemoglobin (HbA1c) <7%.[8]
- Optimizing weight in obese and lean—obesity is associated with both infertility and several adverse pregnancy outcomes including birth defects. Underweight women (especially those with eating disorders) have a 20% increase in risk for preterm birth and a 40% increase in risk of having a small for gestational age infant in one large cohort study.[9]
- Replacement of teratogenic drugs such as angiotensin-converting-enzyme (ACE) inhibitors, angiotensin receptor

blockers (ARBs), statins, lithium, valproic acid, streptomycin, tetracycline, and methotrexate by safer alternatives few months before pregnancy.

PRECONCEPTION CARE FOR HIGH-RISK WOMEN WITH CHRONIC MEDICAL DISORDERS[10]

Women with chronic medical disorders can benefit to a great extent with preconception counseling and interventions which can work to make their pregnancies much safer for them and also improves the perinatal outcome. Some important conditions are discussed briefly further:

- *Diabetes:* Preconceptional advice on diet, exercise, and weight loss is crucial for good outcome. Women should be explained that with good glycemic control, the risks of miscarriage, congenital malformations, stillbirth, and neonatal death is reduced. ADA recommends an A1c of <7% before planning pregnancy. Women with higher levels are at an increased risk of miscarriage and teratogenesis. Self-monitoring of blood glucose and management of hypoglycemic symptoms should be explained.
- *Hypertension:* The goal should be to control blood pressure prior to conception. ACE inhibitors should be stopped before pregnancy (fetal growth restriction, oligohydramnios, and renal failure in fetus) and replaced by safer alternatives. Methyldopa or labetalol are the drugs of choice in pregnancy. Those with chronic hypertension should be assessed for end-organ damage (heart, eye, and kidney) and referred to the concerned specialist.
- *Asthma:* Women should be advised to use their peak flow meters regularly. Those with repeated asthmatic attacks or severe disease should be referred to a specialist in asthma therapy and not managed by the local doctor. If necessary, the use of steroids (inhaled and systemic) in pregnancy is generally safe as compared to the risk of maternal acid-base disturbances and fetal hypoxemia.
- *Cardiac disease:* Women with a history of cardiac problems should be referred to a cardiologist for baseline cardiac assessments and discussion of potential pregnancy risks. Risk assessment of the women is done by the modified World Health Organization (WHO) classification. Women who fall in the WHO Class III and IV should be counseled against pregnancy and the appropriate contraception should be offered.
- *Epilepsy:* Women should be referred to a neurologist for a thorough discussion of the risk of anticonvulsant medications, adjustment of drug regimen, and close monitoring during pregnancy.

  Polytherapy should be avoided to minimize the teratogenic effects of anticonvulsants. In particular, valproate should be discontinued if seizures can be adequately controlled with an alternative drug, since valproate appears to be a more potent teratogen than other antiepileptic drugs. Preconceptional folic acid (4 mg/day) is advised for women on anticonvulsants.
- *Chronic renal disease:* Women should be informed that the outcome of pregnancy and any adverse effects on underlying renal disease are influenced by the presence and degree of renal impairment, hypertension (10% risk of fetal loss if preexisting), and proteinuria. Renal disease during pregnancy is associated with risk of prematurity, growth

restriction, and deterioration in maternal renal function.

Women with renal transplants should be asked to avoid pregnancy for a minimum of 2 years until renal function is optimized on a reduced amount of immunosuppressants.

- *Thyroid disorders:* Routine screening of thyroid function and antibodies in women planning a pregnancy is advisable. Severe and untreated thyrotoxicosis should prompt referral to an endocrinologist during the preconceptional period, as this condition can lead to anovulation, miscarriage, growth restriction, and preterm delivery. In newly diagnosed hypothyroidism, specialist advice should be sought about the levothyroxine starting dose.
- *Systemic lupus erythematosus:* The prognosis is best when the disease has been quiescent for at least 6 months prior to pregnancy and the patient's underlying renal function is stable and normal or near normal. Maternal medications may need to be changed because of potential fetal risks.
- *Inherited thrombophilias:* These women are at higher risk of thromboembolic complications during pregnancy because of pregnancy-associated changes in several coagulation factors; in some cases, they are at increased risk of adverse pregnancy outcome as well. Indications for and management of anticoagulation should be addressed with a thrombosis specialist.
- *Dental caries* and other oral diseases (e.g., periodontal disease) are common and may be associated with pregnancy complications, such as preterm delivery; thus, referral to a dentist is essential.

TERATOGENESIS[11,12]

The study of birth defects and their etiology is called teratology. A teratogen is an agent that acts during embryonic or fetal development to produce a permanent alteration of form and function causing structural abnormalities. It acts by producing cell death, altering normal growth of tissues, or interfering with normal cellular differentiation or other morphologic processes. It can result in fetal death, fetal growth restriction, birth defects, and impaired neurological development. Hadegen is an agent that interferes with normal maturation and function of an organ, while trophogen is an agent that alters growth.

Hadegen and trophogen typically affect in fetal or perinatal period, thus, are fetotoxins rather than teratogens.

Characteristics of Teratogen

A teratogen may be a drug, a maternal disease, a chemical, infectious agent, or a physical agent. For an agent to act as a teratogen, it must have the following characteristics:

- The agent must cross placenta.
- Exposure must occur during critical developmental period.
- The abnormality should have been completely characterized, preferably done by a geneticist or a dysmorphologist.
- Epidemiological findings must be consistent.
- The suspected teratogen must cause defect in animal studies.

Teratogenicity

The teratogenic effect that an agent will have depends on a few factors.

- *Route of exposure:* For instance, a drug given by systemic route may have more teratogenic effect than a dermal or local application of the same drug, e.g., isotretinoin.

- *Dose of the teratogen:* The teratogenic effects are directly related to the dose of teratogen administered. The same agent in smaller doses may not cause any teratogenic effect. Similarly, very high doses of an agent may result in cell death, thus, not causing an teratogenic effect.
- Peak effect of the teratogen.
- *Genetic predisposition:* Certain individuals may be more susceptible to a teratogen than others.
- Sex of the fetus.
- *Species:* An agent which is teratogenic in one species may not have the same effect in the others. A classic example of this is thalidomide. This drug is teratogenic in humans but not in mice.

Timing of Teratogenic Effects and the Critical Developmental Period

It is important to know the important stages of development of various organ systems. A teratogenic exposure during these critical periods cause maximum effect. **Figure 1** shows the periods of organogenesis in the human fetus. The black bars represent critical period of organ development. An exposure of a teratogen at this period can result in major structural defects. The rest of the bar, however, represents the period of cell differentiation. An exposure at this time causes only minor malformation or fetal growth restriction or functional dysfunction.

All-or-none effect: A significant exposure that occurs during the first 10–14 days after fertilization may result in cell death.

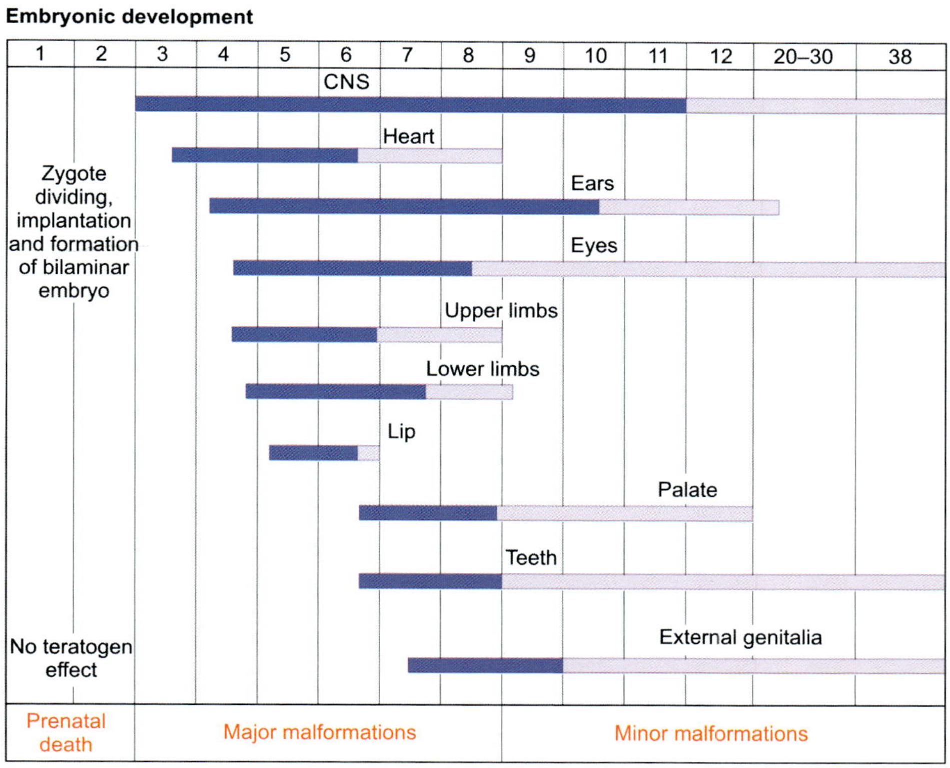

Fig. 1: Critical periods of organ development. (CNS: central nervous system)

Spontaneous abortion may occur if there is death of enough number of cells. However, when only some cells are damaged, then their roles may be compensated by other cells. This is known as the all-or-none theory. For instance, an early significant exposure to radiation results in either pregnancy loss or no abnormalities at all.

Counseling for Medication Exposure

Presenting risk information: It should cover embryonic, fetal risks during drug exposure, and also risks and/or genetic implications of the condition for which the drug being administered. The risks associated with not treating the condition should be explained.

Pregnancy and lactation labeling rules (PLLR): The pregnancy and lactation labeling rule or PLLR has deleted the categories of letters and now contains more comprehensive information about the potential risks and benefits to the pregnant lady and her fetus due to the drug. It also describes how the risk will be different at various trimesters of pregnancy. This can be useful for counseling after an exposure.

Drug classification for therapeutic guidance for prescription in pregnancy.

Teratogens[11]

Alcohol[13]

The prevalence of alcohol use during pregnancy is 9.8% globally. Alcohol is a potent teratogen. It is estimated that 1 in every 67 women consuming alcohol will develop fetal alcohol syndrome. The criteria for documented prenatal alcohol exposure are:

- *Fetal alcohol spectrum disorders (FASD):* The updated institute of management (IOM) has defined diagnostic criteria for the various FASD. The different FASD have been elaborated upon in **Table 1**.

Hence, alcohol is known to cause all these disorders which are preventable. There is no safe trimester and no safe known limit of alcohol consumption during pregnancy. At-risk pregnant women should be identified and counseled about the effects of alcohol preconceptionally and at-booking visit play an important role in preventing alcohol-related disorders. **Table 2** represents some of the common teratogens and their effects.

TABLE 1: Diagnostic criteria for fetal alcohol spectrum disorders.

Disorder	*Documented prenatal alcohol exposure*	*Clinical features*
Fetal alcohol syndrome (FAS)	±	*Requires all features, A–D:* A. *A characteristic pattern of minor facial anomalies, including ≥2 of the following:* (1) Short palpebral fissures; (2) thin vermilion border of the upper lip; and (3) smooth philtrum B. *Prenatal and/or postnatal growth deficiency:* Height and/or weight ≤10th percentile C. *Deficient brain growth, abnormal morphogenesis, or abnormal neurophysiology, including ≥1 of the following:* (1) Head circumference ≤10th percentile; (2) structural brain anomalies; and (3) recurrent nonfebrile seizures (other causes of seizures having been ruled out) D. Neurobehavioral impairment

Contd...

Contd...

Disorder	***Documented prenatal alcohol exposure***	***Clinical features***
Partial fetal alcohol syndrome (PFAS)	±	*Requires features, A–B:* A. *A characteristic pattern of minor facial anomalies, including ≥2 of the following:* (1) Short palpebral fissures; (2) thin vermilion border of the upper lip; and (3) smooth philtrum B. Neurobehavioral impairment
Alcohol-related neurodevelopmental disorder (ARND)	Yes	In children <3 years and neurobehavioral impairment
Alcohol-related birth defects (ARBD)	Yes	*One or more specific major malformations demonstrated in animal models and human studies to be the result of prenatal alcohol exposure:* Cardiac—atrial septal defects, aberrant great vessels, ventricular septal defects, conotruncal heart defects; skeletal—radioulnar synostosis, vertebral segmentation defects, large joint contractures, scoliosis; renal—aplastic/hypoplastic/dysplastic kidneys, "horseshoe" kidneys/ureteral duplications; eyes—strabismus, ptosis, retinal vascular anomalies, optic nerve hypoplasia; ears—conductive hearing loss, neurosensory hearing loss

TABLE 2: Teratogens and their effects.

Drug class	***Mechanism***	***Effects***
Antiepileptic medications		
Valproate	• Highest risk • Mode of action—GABA agonist + glutamate antagonist	Neural tube defects
Phenytoin	Twofold higher risk for malformations	*Fetal hydantoin syndrome:* • Hypertelorism, low nasal bridge • Midface hypoplasia • Hypoplasia of distal phalanges and nails • Growth impairment, intellectual disability
Others: • Phenobarbital • Topiramate		Features similar to fetal hydantoin syndrome
Antihypertensives		
ACE inhibitors Angiotensin receptor blocking agents	Disrupt the fetal renin–angiotensin system	*ACE inhibitor fetopathy:* • Fetal hypotension, renal hypoperfusion with subsequent ischemia and anuria • Fetal growth restriction and calvarium maldevelopment • Pulmonary hypoplasia or limb contractures

Contd...

Contd...

Drug class	***Mechanism***	***Effects***
Antifungals		
Fluconazole	• Inhibit lanosterol 14-alpha demethylase CYP51 • At a dose 400–800 mg daily in first trimester	*Malformations resembling Antley–Bixler syndrome:* • Trapezoidocephaly • Mid face hypoplasia • Cartilage abnormalities • Multiple synostoses • Skeletal fractures
Anti-inflammatory		
Indomethacin	NSAID	• Constriction of fetal ductus arteriosus and subsequent pulmonary hypertension (if taken for more than 3 days) • Decreased fetal urine production and amniotic fluid volume • Bronchopulmonary hypoplasia • Intraventricular hemorrhage • Necrotizing enterocolitis
Aspirin	• Low dose of 100 mg daily or less does not confer for malformations • High dose in third trimester should be avoided	• Cleft lip and palate • Spina bifida • Diaphragmatic hernia • Cardiac defects
Leflunomide	A pyrimidine synthesis inhibitor for rheumatoid arthritis	Hydrocephalus, eye anomalies, skeletal anomalies
Antimicrobials		
Nitrofurantoin		• Cleft lip (1 case per 1,000) • Hypoplastic left heart syndrome (<1 per 1,000) • Hemolytic anemia in glucose 6 phosphate dehydrogenase (G6PD) deficiency
Sulfonamides		• Esophageal atresia or diaphragmatic hernia—1 per 1,000 cases • Hemolytic anemia in G6PD deficiency • Neonatal jaundice—displace bilirubin from protein-binding sites
Tetracyclines		Yellowish-brown discoloration of deciduous teeth if used after 25 weeks gestation
Antineoplastic agents		
Methotrexate	• Folic acid antagonist vulnerable at 8–10 weeks postconception	*Fetal methotrexate–aminopterin syndrome:* • Craniosynostosis with a clover leaf skull • Wide nasal bridge

Contd...

Contd...

Drug class	***Mechanism***	***Effects***
	• Threshold dose 10 mg/week • Standard 50 mg/m^2 dose given to treat ectopic pregnancy or induce abortion exceeds the threshold dose	• Low set ears • Micrognathia • Limb anomalies • CNS and cardiac defects
Trastuzumab	Monoclonal antibody against HER2 used in breast and gastric cancer	Oligohydramnios resulting in pulmonary hypoplasia, renal failure, skeletal abnormalities
Cyclophosphamide	Alkylating agent	• Spontaneous abortions among healthcare workers • Skeletal, limb, cleft palate, eye abnormalities
Tamoxifen	Selective estrogen receptor modulator used in breast cancer	Ambiguous genitalia and craniofacial anomalies
Antipsychotics		
Lithium	Prevalence is 1–4 per 1,000 exposed pregnancies *Neonatal lithium toxicity:* • Occurs due to exposure near delivery • Therefore, dosage should be decreased or discontinued 2–3 days prior to delivery • Findings may persist for 2 weeks	*Neonatal lithium toxicity:* • Arrythmias • Hypoglycemia • Nephrogenic diabetes insipidus • Floppy infant syndrome (hypotonia, respiratory distress, bradycardia, cyanosis, feeding difficulties)
Retinoids	• Mode of action—inhibit neural crest cell migration causing cranial neural crest defects • Dose—more than 10,000 IU per day in first trimester of retinol	*Retinoic acid embryopathy:* • Ventriculomegaly • Maldevelopment of facial bones • Microtia or anotia • Cleft palate • Conotruncal heart defects • Thymic aplasia or hypoplasia
Thyroid medications		
Methimazole		• Aplasia cutis congenita (full-thickness skin defect including underlying bone) • Choanal atresia • Esophageal atresia

Contd...

Contd...

Drug class	***Mechanism***	***Effects***
Radioiodine		• Fetal and neonatal hypothyroidism leading to decreased mental capacity and delayed skeletal maturation • Pregnancy should be avoided for 6–12 months following treatment
Thalidomide	• Cause malformations in 20% fetus exposed between 34 and 50 days menstrual age • Timing of exposure may be closely related to type of defect	*Phocomelia:* • Limb reduction defects—absence or underdevelopment of one or more long bones • Cardiac defects • GI defects • External ear and eye defects
Warfarin	• Vitamin K antagonist • Embryopathy result from exposure between 6 and 9 weeks gestation with a prevalence of 6%	*Fetal warfarin syndrome:* • Nasal hypoplasia and choanal atresia • Stippled epiphysis of femur, humerus, calcanei, distal phalanges • CNS anomalies—agenesis of corpus callosum, vermian agenesis • Optic atrophy • Deafness
Substance abuse		
Cocaine	CNS stimulant vasoconstrictive and hypertensive effects	• Maternal complications—cerebrovascular hemorrhage, myocardial damage, placental abruption • Fetal complications—cleft palate, microcephaly, FGR/IUGR, preterm births, behavioral abnormalities, and cognitive impairments in later life
Cannabinoids	• Most common recreational drug in pregnancy worldwide • Disinhibition of dopaminergic neurons, resulting from presynaptic inhibition of GABA neurons	Neurodevelopmental abnormalities, e.g., decreased attention span and poor visual–motor coordination
Methamphetamine	• Prescribed to treat narcolepsy and ADHDs • Sympathomimetic amine derived from dextroamphetamine enhances dopamine release and blocks its uptake	Not considered teratogenic but associated with SGA births and children at risks for developmental delays and behavioral abnormalities

Contd...

Contd...

Drug class	*Mechanism*	*Effects*
Opioids	Inhibition of neuro-transmitter release	Preterm births, FGR, fetal death, placental abruption, neonatal narcotic withdrawal (neonatal abstinence syndrome) (40–90% of exposed newborns), central nervous system irritability, feeding difficulties, failure to thrive
Tobacco	• Cross placenta • Nicotine stimulates presynaptic acety-lcholine receptors and enhances ACh release and metabolism	• Orofacial clefts, congenital defects, growth restriction, low birth weight, preterm labor, sudden fetal death, • Placenta previa, abruption
Toluene		Fetal embryopathy
Radiation exposure		
	<50 mGy (<5 rads). Radiation exposure in one plain X-ray: 0.01–10 rads (lumbar spine)	• *0–2 weeks:* None, or spontaneous abortion • *>2 weeks:* Subtle effect
	50–100 mGy. Radiation exposure in a CT scan of pelvis: 50 rads	• *2–25 weeks:* Teratogenic; congenital abnormalities, microcephaly, mental retardation, growth restriction. Maximum between 8 and 15 weeks • *>25 weeks:* No teratogenic effect at diagnostic doses of <100 mGy
	100–500 mGy	Decision to abort
	>500 mGy (>50 rads)	Potentially teratogenic and considerable fetal damage

(ACE: angiotensin-converting enzyme; ACh: acetylcholine; ADHDs: attention-deficit/hyperactivity disorders; CNS: central nervous system; FGR/IUGR: fetal growth restriction/intrauterine growth restriction; GABA: gamma-amino butyric acid; GI: gastrointestinal; HER2: human epidermal growth factor receptor 2; NSAID: nonsteroidal anti-inflammatory drug; SGA: small for gestational age)

REFERENCES

1. Johnson K, Posner SF, Biermann J, Cordero JF, Atrash HK, Parker CS, et al. Recommendations to improve Preconceptional Health and Health care. MMWR Recomm Rep. 2006;55:1.
2. Atrash H, Jack BW, Johnson K, Coonrod DV, Moos MK, Stubblefield PG, et al. Where is "W"oman in MCH? Am J Obstet Gynecol. 2008;199:S259-65.
3. Jack BW, Atrash H, Coonrod DV, Moos MK, O'Donnell J, Johnson K. The clinical content of preconceptional care: an overview and preparation of this supplement. Am J Obstet Gynecol. 2008;199:S266-79.
4. Farahi N, Zolotor A. Recommendations for preconception Counseling and Care. Am Fam Physician. 2013;88(8):499-506.
5. Dean SV, Lassi ZS, Imam AM, Bhutta ZA. Preconception care: promoting reproductive planning. Reprod Health. 2014;11(Suppl 3):S2.
6. https://www.fogsi.org/gcpr-preconception-care [Last accessed March, 2024].
7. MoHFW 2018. Anemia Mukt Bharat: intensified – National Iron Plus Initiative:

operational guidelines for program managers, Ministry of Health and Family Welfare, Government of India, New Delhi. [Last accessed March, 2024].

8. American Diabetes Association. Management of diabetes in pregnancy. Diabetes Care. 2015;38 Suppl:S77-9.
9. Tabet M, Flick LH, Tuuli MG, Macones GA, Chang JJ. Prepregnancy body mass index in a first uncomplicated pregnancy and outcomes of a second pregnancy. Am J Obstet Gynecol. 2015;213(4):548.e1.
10. Sackey JA, Blazey-Martin D. (2015). The preconception office visit. [online] Available from https://sso.uptodate.com/contents/the-preconception-office-visit/print [Last accessed March, 2024].
11. Cunningham FG, Leveno K, Dashe J, Hoffman B, Spong C, Casey B. Williams Obstetrics, 26th edition. Columbus, OH: McGraw-Hill Education; 2022.
12. Resnik R, Creasy RK, Iams JD, Lockwood CJ, Moore T, Greene MF. Creasy and Resnik's Maternal-Fetal Medicine: Principles and Practice, 7th edition. Philadelphia: WB Saunders; 2013.
13. Hur YM, Choi J, Park S, Oh SS, Kim YJ. Prenatal maternal alcohol exposure: diagnosis and prevention of fetal alcohol syndrome. Obstet Gynecol Sci. 2022;65(5):385-94.

2

CHAPTER

Antenatal Screening for Fetal Aneuploidies

Sangeeta Gupta, Harshiba Kaur

KEY POINTS

1. Aneuploidies are major causes of perinatal mortality and childhood morbidity.
2. The most common autosomal and sex chromosome aneuploidies are trisomies of chromosome 21, 18, 13, and monosomy of chromosome X.
3. Prenatal screening for aneuploidies should be offered universally after providing adequate and appropriate counseling.
4. There is a plethora of tests available for screening of aneuploidies with varying detection rates (DR).
5. Invasive testing, including amniocentesis and chorionic villus sampling (CVS), remains the diagnostic testing for aneuploidy detection.
6. Since these invasive tests have an inherent albeit small risk of miscarriage, they cannot be offered in all pregnancies.
7. It is hence important to correctly counsel the couple regarding the choice of aneuploidy screening tests which will help the clinicians to select the woman who that require invasive testing.

INTRODUCTION

Aneuploidy is the presence of one or more extra chromosomes or the absence of one or more chromosomes. It is more common in women with advanced maternal age (except Turner syndrome) but can affect fetuses of mothers of any age; hence, screening for risk of aneuploidies should be offered after counseling, universally in all pregnancies.

Chromosomal abnormalities affect approximately 1 in 150 pregnancies and are responsible for 50% of early pregnancy losses.[1] The effects of aneuploidy may range from incompatible with life to intellectual and physical disability. The aim of screening tests is to detect aneuploid fetuses that are compatible with survival beyond the period of viability. The common aneuploidies that would be discussed here are trisomy 21 [Down syndrome (DS)], trisomy 18 (Edwards syndrome), and trisomy 13 (Patau syndrome).

The risk of aneuploidies increases with maternal age and decreases with gestational age (30% of trisomy 21 fetuses and 80% of trisomies 13 and 18 fetuses die in utero between 12 weeks and term). Turner syndrome is unrelated to maternal age, and the prevalence is 1 in 1,500 at 12 weeks and 1 in 4,000 at 40 weeks. Other sex chromosomal aneuploidies are also unrelated to maternal age and their rate of fetal death is similar to the euploid fetuses (47, XXY, 47, XXX).

SCREENING FOR CHROMOSOMAL ANEUPLOIDIES

The screening for fetal aneuploidies has undergone dramatic changes in the past few decades. In the 1960s, the two criteria (maternal age >35 years and family history) were the traditional risk factors for offering diagnostic testing (amniocentesis and karyotyping). Unfortunately, these criteria have proven to be poor screening tools for DS, exposing 15–20% of pregnant women to invasive testing, with its inherent pregnancy loss rate, while detecting only 30–35% of affected pregnancies. There has been inclusion of second-trimester biochemistries in the 1980s followed by first-trimester biochemistries and fetal ultrasound in the 1990s. The most recent advancement for screening has been cell-free fetal deoxyribonucleic acid (cffDNA) in maternal blood [noninvasive prenatal screening (NIPS)].

Prenatal screening for aneuploidies should be offered to all women after providing necessary information regarding the sensitivity, false-positive rates (FPRs), limitations, and turnaround time. This should be done irrespective of age or risk of chromosomal aneuploidies. Nonetheless, the choice of the test chosen will depend upon the obstetric and family history, presence of anyone with intellectual disability or a genetic diagnosis in the family, multiple miscarriages, gestational age, and the number of fetuses. The pretest counseling should be done in a clear, effective, and nondirective manner and allow the patient enough time to understand and make an informed decision. Multiple screening tests should not be performed simultaneously. Post-test counseling is necessary regardless of the result of the screening test. If negative, the couple should be informed of the residual risk, which is the chance that the fetus may still have a chromosomal abnormality, depending on the detection rate of the test and the condition targeted for testing.[2] If screen positive, counseling should be provided regarding the positive predictive value of the screening test, and diagnostic test which should be offered depending upon the gestational age after appropriate genetic counseling.

First-trimester Screening

The serum biochemistry and ultrasound markers have been used for aneuploidy screening for many years. Determination of correct gestational age is essential and integral for calculation of accurate risk calculation. The multiples of median (MoM) of serum biochemistry and the centiles of nuchal translucency (NT) alter with gestational age. Hence, serum biochemistry samples should be preferably drawn after the first-trimester scan done from 11 weeks to 13 weeks 6 days. The ultrasound should be performed as per the Fetal Medicine Foundation (FMF) guidelines by accredited sonographers. Similarly, serum biochemistry is also performed in accredited laboratories with strict quality control. The software used for calculation of risks should be validated (common software used are life-cycle and Kryptor).

Serum Biochemistry

These are biochemical tests done in maternal serum. The dual marker is the most recommended, performed in the first trimester between 9 weeks and 13 weeks 6 days and includes estimation of the free beta-human chorionic gonadotropin (beta-hCG) and the pregnancy-associated plasma protein A (PAPP-A). The hCG is a glycoprotein that is produced by the developing embryo and later by the placenta. PAPP-A is a complex high-molecular-weight glycoprotein which is also a placental product. In pregnancies affected by DS, the measured beta hGC is high and PAPP-A is low. The raw values are converted to MoM as per the gestational age. **Table 1** depicts the variation of MoMs of the two biochemical markers in different aneuploidies. The calculation of risk is done

TABLE 1: Expected biochemistry levels in euploid and aneuploid fetuses.[4,5]

Study population	Median-free beta-hCG (MoM)	Median PAPP-A (MoM)
Euploid	1.0	1.0
Trisomy 21	2.0	0.5
Trisomy 18	0.2	0.2
Trisomy 13	0.5	0.3
Turner syndrome	1.0	0.4

(hCG: human chorionic gonadotropin; MoM: multiple of median; PAPP-A: pregnancy-associated plasma protein A)

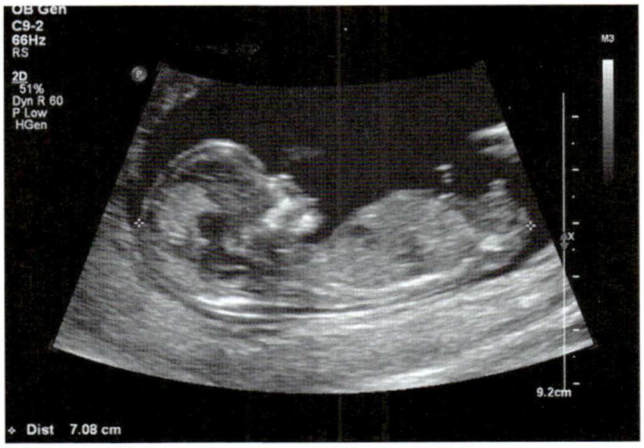

Fig. 1: Crown–rump length.

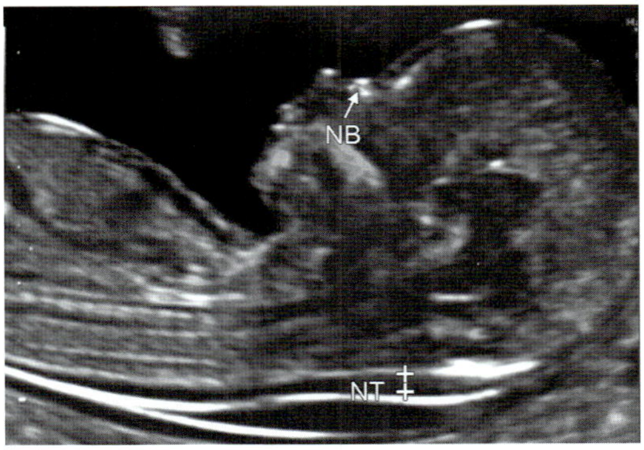

Fig. 2: Normal nuchal translucency (NT). (NB: nasal bone)

by using appropriate software wherein maternal age, maternal weight, ethnicity, smoking, type of conception, gestational age, number of fetuses, and chorionicity determine a priori risk and adjustments are made in PAPP-A and beta-hCG for calculation of MoMs. This adjustment is necessary for accurate risk calculation.[3] Combining the dual marker with an appropriately measured NT has a DR of 85% with a FPR of 5% for DS.

There is evidence that the "first-trimester quadruple marker" by addition of placental growth factor (PlGF) and alpha fetoprotein (AFP) helps to further bring down the FPR to 1–1.5% and improves the detection rate to almost 98%. The additional advantage of adding PlGF is the detection of early onset preeclampsia (requiring delivery before 34 weeks). The women who are screen positive for preeclampsia can be given aspirin to reduce the incidence of early onset preeclampsia by 80%.

First-trimester Ultrasound

The ultrasound is performed between 11 weeks and 13 weeks 6 days. The objective of this ultrasound examination is to check for number of fetuses, chorionicity in case of multiple pregnancy, determination of gestational age [measurement of crown–rump length (CRL) **(Fig. 1)**], check viability and markers of aneuploidy [NT, nasal bone (NB), tricuspid regurgitation (TR), and ductus venosus (DV)]. Uterine artery doppler is also done in the same sitting which is an important marker of preeclampsia screening. At the end of the first trimester, the scan also offers an opportunity to detect gross fetal abnormalities. As mentioned earlier, the ultrasound should be performed as per the FMF guidelines by accredited sonographers.

The NT refers to the fluid-filled space on the dorsal aspect of the fetal neck **(Fig. 2)**. CRL range should be a minimum 45 mm and maximum 84 mm for the measurement of NT.

The NT measurement must be precise and should be carried out by certified sonologists as even an undermeasurement of 0.5 mm may decrease the sensitivity of risk detection by 18%.

Nuchal Translucency: Increased Nuchal Translucency and its Associations

The NT is a function of CRL and increases with increasing CRL. There are nomograms available, which must be referred to for defining an NT that is >95th percentile for a given CRL **(Fig. 3)**. A cutoff of NT >3.5 mm is taken as >99th percentile for all CRLs.

The risk of adverse fetal outcomes is directly proportional to the degree of NT enlargement. A high NT of 3.5 mm or more may be indicative of many other conditions besides chromosomal aneuploidies like cardiac defects, skeletal dysplasias, genetic syndromes, single gene defects and an active search for pathologies must be undertaken if aneuploidies are not found in these cases. This is done by detailed anomaly evaluation, further genetic testing in the form of chromosomal microarray analysis (CMA) and whole exome sequencing (depending upon personal and family history), fetal echo, and evaluation for fetal infections.

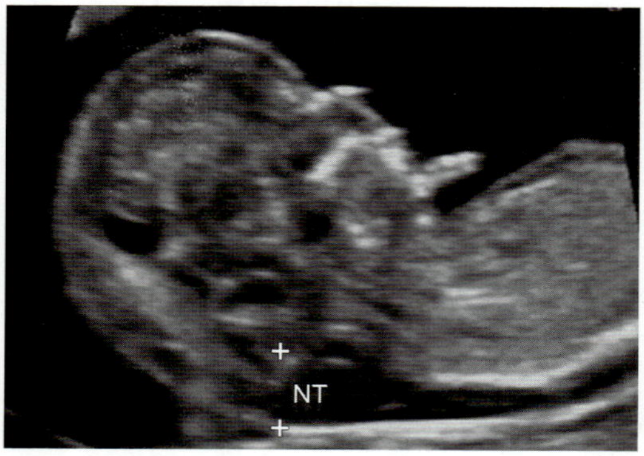

Fig. 3: Increased nuchal translucency (NT).

When NT alone is used to modify the age-based risk, the DR for DS is 70%.

In trisomies 18 and 13, other ultrasound findings can be appreciated beside increased NT in the first-trimester ultrasound. Trisomies 18 and 13 are observed in about 65% of fetuses with holoprosencephaly, 55% with exomphalos, and 30% with megacystis. Absence of the NB, abnormal flow in the DV, and TR are observed in about 50%, 55%, and 30%, respectively, of fetuses with trisomies 18 and 13.[6]

Combined First-trimester Screening

Combined first-trimester screening (cFTS) is the most accepted method of screening for aneuploides currently and most widely recommended by most of the guidelines.[7] The addition of maternal factors, serum biochemistry, and ultrasound markers helps to improve the DR and bring down the FPR; e.g., combining maternal age, NT, NB, and dual marker gives a DR of 90% with a FPR of 3% for trisomy 21. Addition of other markers such as wave of DV and TR further improve the DR to 93%.[8]

Second-trimester Screening

Serum Biochemistry

The triple or quadruple marker can be used in the second trimester from 15 0/7 weeks to 20 6/7 weeks of gestation (the gestational age range for screening varies among different laboratories). This can be used in women who present late or have missed their first-trimester screening.

Earlier triple marker which consisted of consisting of beta-hCG, AFP, and unconjugated estriol in addition to maternal factors like age, weight, race, and the presence of pregestational diabetes was being used. It has a low DR of 60–65% and is no more recommended. Quadruple marker consists of the addition of dimeric inhibin A to the triple marker and has an improved DR of 75–80% with a 5% FPR.[9] AFP may help in detection of women with open neural tube defects, but with the advancement of technology, ultrasound remains the mainstay for their diagnosis with a DR of up to 100%. Some laboratories offer the Penta test, which adds hyperglycosylated hCG to the quadruple test. One retrospective review showed improved second-trimester screening with the Penta test, but it is needed further prospective trials for the same.[10]

No second-trimester screening should be offered after a standard cFTS is performed: The first trimester and quad should not be performed in an unlinked manner or else as they might give an exceptionally high false-positive result or provide contradictory risk estimations.

Second-trimester Ultrasonography

The ultrasonographic findings in DS are commonly very subtle and are known as soft markers, unlike those in trisomies of chromosome 18 and 13. Soft markers are not structural anomalies but are ultrasound findings that are found more frequently in aneuploid as compared to euploid fetuses. The various soft markers are ventriculomegaly, increased nuchal fold thickness, absent or hypoplastic NB, aberrant right subclavian artery, short-long bones, echogenic bowel, and mild hydronephrosis. Each of these markers has a different likelihood ratio and is used for the calculation of risk of DS in the anomaly scan done at 18–22 weeks and multiplying it with a priori risk based on maternal age and biochemical screening. Other findings can be increased frontomaxillary angle, clinodactyly, and sandal gap. However, the DR of second-trimester ultrasound alone for DS is poor (60% detection). Hence, women who present in the second trimester should be offered a quadruple marker for screening for DS.

In trisomy 18, there is a cluster of classical ultrasound findings, namely microcephaly, strawberry-shaped skull, Dandy–Walker malformation, choroid plexus cysts, absent corpus callosum, meningomyelocele, facial clefts, major cardiovascular defects, omphalocele, diaphragmatic hernia, single umbilical artery, renal anomalies, radial aplasia, clenched fists/overlapping fingers, and club feet/rocker bottom feet, in the second trimester and are almost never isolated. Early onset fetal growth restriction (FGR) is the most common abnormality reported in these fetuses. This may or may not be associated with polyhydramnios.

Trisomy 13 may present with microcephaly, hypotelorism, cleft lip and palate, cardiovascular defects, omphalocele, echogenic kidneys, polydactyly, and early onset FGR.

Table 2 depicts the performance of different methods of screening for aneuploidies.

NONINVASIVE PRENATAL SCREENING

Noninvasive prenatal test (NIPT) has emerged as one of the best performing screening tools for aneuploidies. Maternal plasma contains small fragments of cell-free fetal (or more accurately placental) DNA which arises from the apoptosis of trophoblastic cells. Up to 10–15% of the cell-free DNA in the maternal plasma is of fetal origin. NIPS uses various sequencing technologies to calculate an extra dosage of chromosomal material in this cffDNA. This test should be performed any

TABLE 2: Performance of different methods of screening for aneuploidies.

Screening test	Detection rate (%)	False-positive rate (%)
MA	30	5
MA + serum free β-hCG and PAPP-A	60–70	5
MA + fetal NT	75–80	5
MA + NT + free β-hCG and PAPP-A (combined test)	85–95	5
Combined test + nasal bone or tricuspid flow or ductus venosus flow	93–96	2.5
MA + serum AFP, free β-hCG, uE3, inhibin A (quadruple test)	70–75	5

(AFP: alpha fetoprotein; hCG: human chorionic gonadotropin; MA: maternal age; NT: nuchal translucency; PAPP-A: pregnancy-associated plasma protein A; uE3: unconjugated estriol)

time after 10 weeks of gestation and requires a minimum fetal fraction of 4% for predicting the risk accurately. Dating, viability, number of fetuses, presence of a vanishing twin, and structural abnormalities should be confirmed by ultrasound before offering NIPS. Maternal factors like high body mass index (BMI) and early gestational age may reduce the fetal fraction and lead to a "no call" report. Although the possibility of aneuploidy is also high (about 60–70%) with a "no call" result, the decision to perform a repeat NIPS versus invasive testing should be individualized. The DR of NIPS is reported as 99.2% with a FPR of 0.09% for trisomy 21. The performance of NIPS for various aneuploidies is shown in **Table 3**. The turnaround time is around 7–10 days. Nonetheless, NIPS remains a screening test and a high-risk result should be confirmed with invasive tests like chorionic villus sampling or amniocentesis. Pregnancies should not be terminated solely

TABLE 3: Performance of NIPS for detection of common aneuploidies.[11]

Condition	Detection rate (%)	FPR (%)
Trisomy 21	99.7	0.04
Trisomy 18	98.2	0.05
Trisomy 13	99.0	0.04
Monosomy X	95.8	0.14
Other sex chromosomal abnormalities	100	0.004

(FPR: false positive rate; NIPS: noninvasive prenatal screening)

based on a high-risk NIPS report. Despite its advantages, NIPS is not a replacement for a good first-trimester scan. Currently, NIPS is used as a contingent in women with intermediate risk on combined screening—this has markedly decreased the number of invasive tests. Also, care should be taken that NIPS is not performed in pregnancies with structural anomalies. NIPS may result in a false-positive test in mothers with a known mosaicism, malignancy, or organ transplant and should not be offered in these cases.

CONTINGENT SCREENING

There are algorithms provided by the FMF and American College of Obstetricians and Gynecologists (ACOG) depending on the risk obtained on the screening test to reduce the rate of invasive testing as they carry a small inherent risk of miscarriage. In this screening, the risk is classified as low, intermediate, or high as per the FMF criteria. Pregnancies with a high-risk screen result (>1:100) should be offered invasive testing directly. Those with an intermediate risk (1:100–1:1,000) should be offered NIPS (after a fetal medicine/genetic opinion), and those with a low risk (<1:1,000) are reassured called for a routine anomaly scan at 18–20 weeks[7] **(Flowchart 1)**.

Flowchart 1: Contingent screening.

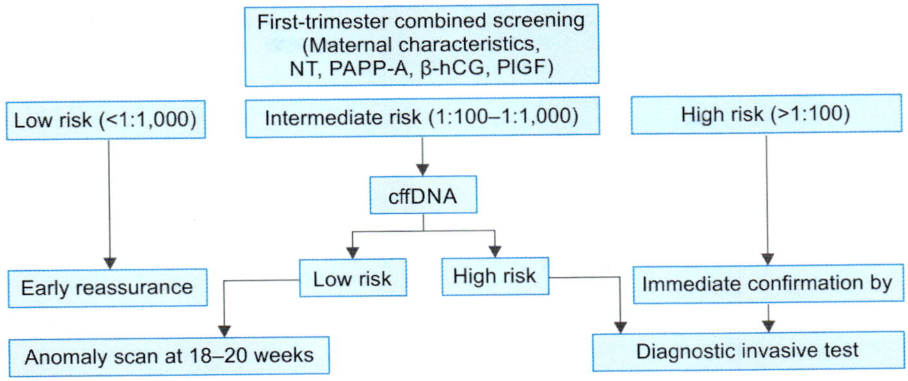

(cffDNA: cell-free deoxyribonucleic acid; hCG: human chorionic gonadotropin; NT: nuchal translucency; PAPP-A: pregnancy-associated plasma protein A; PIGF: placental growth factor)

INVASIVE TESTING

For the confirmation of a positive screen test, CVS or amniocentesis is performed depending upon the gestational age and the sample (chorionic villous or amniotic fluid) is sent for quantitative fluorescent polymerase chain reaction (QFPCR) (rapid test with a turnaround time of 1–3 days) and G-band karyotyping (that may require culture and takes up to 2–3 weeks). Screen positive results may be associated with chromosomal abnormalities other than aneuploidies, like microdeletions and duplications, and hence microarray is preferred over conventional karyotyping which can detect microscopic changes in the chromosomal structure. The drawback of microarray is that it may not pick up balanced translocations.

Five percent of trisomy 18 fetuses may have a confined placental mosaicism, where the placenta may have a normal karyotype. Hence, the preferred diagnostic test is amniocentesis over CVS when this is suspected.

The recurrence risk should also be explained. In free trisomies (due to nondisjunction), the risk is less than 1%. In case of translocation trisomies, a parental karyotype must be done. If the unbalanced translocation is of maternal origin, then the risk of occurrence is 15%. When the father is the translocation carrier, then the risk is 5%.[2] This warrants referral for genetic counseling.

REFERENCES

1. Committee on Practice Bulletins—Obstetrics, Committee on Genetics, and the Society for Maternal-Fetal Medicine. Practice bulletin no. 163: screening for fetal aneuploidy. Obstet Gynecol. 2016;127(5):e123-37.
2. Counseling about genetic testing and communication of genetic test results. Committee Opinion No. 693. American College of Obstetricians and Gynecologists. Obstet Gynecol. 2017;129:771-2.
3. Kagan KO, Wright D, Spencer K, Molina FS, Nicolaides KH. First-trimester screening for trisomy 21 by free beta-human chorionic gonadotropin and pregnancy-associated plasma protein-A: impact of maternal and pregnancy characteristics. Ultrasound Obstet Gynecol. 2008;31(5):493-502.
4. Wagner P, Sonek J, Hoopmann M, Abele H, Kagan KO. First-trimester screening for trisomies 18 and 13, triploidy and Turner syndrome by detailed early anomaly scan. Ultrasound Obstet Gynecol. 2016;48(4):446-51.

5. Kagan KO, Sonek J, Wagner P, Hoopmann M. Principles of first trimester screening in the age of noninvasive prenatal diagnosis: screening for chromosomal abnormalities. Arch Gynecol Obstet. 2017;296(4):645-51.
6. Kagan KO, Cicero S, Staboulidou I, Wright D, Nicolaides KH. Fetal nasal bone in screening for trisomies 21, 18 and 13 and Turner syndrome at 11–13 weeks of gestation. Ultrasound Obstet Gynecol. 2009b;33:259-64.
7. American College of Obstetricians and Gynecologists' Committee on Practice Bulletins—Obstetrics; Committee on Genetics; Society for Maternal-Fetal Medicine. Screening for Fetal Chromosomal Abnormalities: ACOG Practice Bulletin, Number 226. Obstet Gynecol. 2020;136(4): e48-69.
8. Evans MI, Van Decruyes H, Nicolaides KH. Nuchal translucency measurements for first-trimester screening: the "price" of inaccuracy. Fetal Diagn Ther. 2007;22:401-4.
9. Santorum M, Wright D, Syngelaki A, Karagioti N, Nicolaides KH. Accuracy of first-trimester combined test in screening for trisomies 21, 18 and 13. Ultrasound Obstet Gynecol. 2017;49(6):714-20.
10. Malone FD, Canick JA, Ball RH, Nyberg DA, Comstock CH, Bukowski R, et al. First- and Second-Trimester Evaluation of Risk (FASTER) Research Consortium. First-trimester or second-trimester screening, or both, for Down's syndrome. N Engl J Med. 2005;353:2001e11.
11. Gil MM, Accurti V, Santacruz B, Plana MN, Nicolaides KH. Analysis of cell-free DNA in maternal blood in screening for aneuploidies: updated meta-analysis. Ultrasound Obstet Gynecol. 2017;50:302-14.

3

CHAPTER

Screening and Prediction of Preeclampsia

Saloni Kamboj, K Aparna Sharma

KEY POINTS

1. Preeclampsia (PE) is a multisystem disorder which is characterized by new onset of hypertension along with significant proteinuria after 20 weeks' gestation.
2. It typically occurs after 20 weeks of pregnancy, but pathogenesis starts earlier, hence the importance of early screening.
3. PE can be categorized into early onset (delivery before 34 weeks) and late onset (delivery after 34 weeks).
4. Early-onset PE is of particular concern due to its association with neonatal morbidity.
5. There are many screening approaches that can be used in first trimester like by maternal history, maternal biophysical markers, and biochemical markers, but the best approach is using an algorithmic (multimodal) [available free on Fetal Medicine Foundation (FMF) site].
6. Hypertensive disorder of pregnancy (HDP)–gestosis score can be used as an effective and feasible prediction policy for low resource settings.
7. In second trimester, maternal factors with uterine artery Doppler measurements and placental growth factor (PlGF) levels can be used for screening
8. Screening in third trimester can be done by using maternal factors, mean arterial pressure (MAP), uterine artery pulsatility index (UTPI), PlGF, and soluble fms-like tyrosine kinase-1 (sFlt-1) measurements.

INTRODUCTION

Preeclampsia is a multisystem disorder which is characterized by new onset of hypertension along with significant proteinuria after 20 weeks' gestation.[1,2] This disorder affects 2–8% of pregnant women and is one of the leading causes of maternal and perinatal morbidity and mortality.[3,4] PE can cause many maternal adverse effects, including impairment of hepatorenal and coagulation systems and in severe form, it can cause pulmonary edema, eclampsia, brain hemorrhage, etc.[5,6] In fetal complications, fetal growth restriction, preterm birth or stillbirth is seen because of uteroplacental insufficiency.[5,7] Moreover, PE is associated with an increased risk of long-term cardiovascular and chronic diseases in both the mothers and their children from the affected pregnancy.[8] Women with PE are also at elevated risk for chronic hypertension, future cardiovascular disease, stroke, metabolic syndromes, cognitive impairment, and chronic end-stage renal disease later in life.[9,10] It has been proposed to further subclassify PE according to gestational age at delivery because evidence suggests that early- and late-onset disease have different pathophysiologic and etiologic pathways. Early-onset PE is associated with a higher risk of adverse maternal and perinatal outcomes.[11]

NEED FOR SCREENING AND PREDICTION

Preeclampsia can be categorized into early-onset (delivery before 34 weeks) and late-onset (delivery after 34 weeks). Early-onset PE is of particular concern due to its association with neonatal morbidity, primarily prematurity.[12] Identifying high-risk pregnancies for early-onset PE during the first trimester is crucial for implementing preventive measures and reducing the overall disease burden. Screening for PE is vital because there are evidence-based interventions, such as low-dose aspirin, that can mitigate its risk, especially when initiated early in pregnancy.[13-15] Screening also aids in identifying high-risk individuals for closer monitoring throughout the gestation.

DIVERSE SCREENING APPROACHES IN FIRST TRIMESTER

Screening by Maternal History

Professional guidelines recommend taking a comprehensive maternal history at the initial prenatal visit. Factors such as chronic diseases, age, and body mass index (BMI) are considered when assessing the risk of PE. While the sensitivity of screening by maternal history alone is relatively low, it is still recommended by the American College of Obstetricians and Gynecologists (ACOG). Estimated detection rate (DR) of PE requiring delivery before 34 and 37 weeks gestation by maternal history alone is about 51% and 43%, respectively, at false-positive rate (FPR) of 10%[16] **(Table 1)**.

Screening by Maternal Biophysical Markers

Blood Pressure

Women who later develop PE often exhibit higher systolic blood pressure (SBP) and mean arterial pressure even before clinical symptoms manifest. MAP is calculated by adding one third of pulse pressure to the diastolic pressure. It is important to learn the correct method of measurement. It is measured with validated automated devices with women in sitting position with back supported and legs uncrossed. Arms should be well supported at the level of the heart and an appropriate-sized adult cuff (small <22 cm, normal 22–32 cm, or large 33–42 cm) should be used. After rest for 5 minutes, blood pressure (BP) is measured in both arms simultaneously. Two sets of recordings are made at 1-minute intervals. The four sets of SBP and diastolic BP (DBP) measurements are required for input into the risk calculator to calculate MAP. If MAP is added along with maternal factors, the DR of PE goes up to 74% for early PE and 49% for late PE with a FPR of 10%. Also, adding the measurement of

TABLE 1: Risk factors to be considered while taking history in first trimester as per the American College of Obstetricians and Gynecologists (ACOG) 2018.[17]

High risk	*Moderate risk*
• Previous pregnancy with PE • Chronic hypertension • Systemic lupus erythematosus • Type 1 or type 2 diabetes mellitus • Renal disease • Multifetal gestation • Antiphospholipid syndrome	• Nulliparity • Age more than 35 years • Interpregnancy interval >10 years • BMI >30 kg/m^2 • Family history of PE (mother or sister) • History of SGA or adverse outcome • Sociodemographic characteristics (African–American race or low socioeconomic status)

(BMI: body mass index; PE: preeclampsia; SGA: small for gestational age)

BP in second trimester further increases the sensitivity to 84% for early PE and 53% for late PE with a FPR of 10%.[18]

Uterine Artery Dopplers

Uterine artery Doppler assessment in the first trimester can identify increased resistance in the spiral arteries, indicating impaired placental function.[19] It is seen that the uterine artery pulsatility index multiple of median (MoM) is found to be significantly increased at 11–13 week's gestation in women who develop PE.[20] The addition of uterine artery Dopplers to maternal factors improves the DR of PE from to 75% and 55% at FPR of 10% for PE requiring delivery before 34 and 37 weeks gestation.[18,21] Technique of measurement is very important. It is done using a transabdominal sonograph and a sagittal section of the uterus is obtained. Then, cervix is identified first and color flow is put to identify each uterine artery along the side of the cervix and uterus at the level of the internal os. Pulsed wave Doppler is then used to cover the whole vessel and care should be taken to ensure that the angle of insonation is <30°. Three similar consecutive waveforms are obtained and the mean pulsatility index (PI) of the left and right arteries is calculated.[22] It is important to ensure that the peak systolic velocity (PSV) is >60 cm/s **(Fig. 1)**. The value >95th centile for gestational age is abnormal.

Screening by Maternal Biochemical Markers

Various biochemical markers have been investigated for predicting PE, including placental growth factor, pregnancy-associated plasma protein-A (PAPP-A), inhibin-A, activin-A, and others.[23] Both PAPP-A and PlGF have proven useful not only for aneuploidy screening but also for PE prediction. Combining these biochemical markers with maternal factors enhances PE detection. PAPP-A is a syncytiotrophoblast-derived metalloproteinase which plays an important role in placental growth and development. PlGF is a glycosylated dimeric glycoprotein, which is a member of the vascular endothelial growth factor

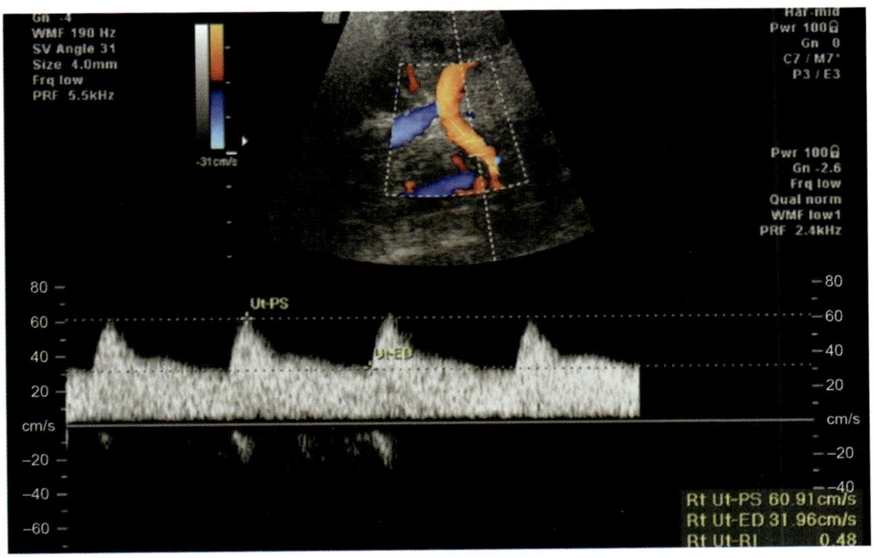

Fig. 1: Measurement of uterine artery pulsatility index (PI).

subfamily. PlGF is proangiogenic and has been speculated to play a role in normal pregnancy and decrease in its level has been implicated in development of PE **(Fig. 2)**. Both PAPP-A and PlGF have shown to be affected by various factors such as gestational age at screening, maternal age maternal weight, racial origin, cigarette smoking, use of assisted reproductive technology (ART) techniques for conception, nulliparity, and preexisting diabetes mellitus. The addition of these biochemical markers to maternal factors improves the DR to 74% and 56%, at FPR of 10%, for PE requiring delivery before 34 and 37 weeks' gestation.[18]

Screening by Maternal Biochemical and Biophysical Markers

Effective screening for PE can be achieved by a combination of maternal factors and biochemical and biophysical markers. Estimated DR of PE requiring delivery before 34 and 37 weeks' gestation in screening by maternal factors with biochemical and biophysical markers are 96% and 77%, respectively, at a FPR of 10%.[18]

Algorithmic Approach: Multimodality

All pregnant women should undergo first-trimester screening for preterm PE using a combined test that incorporates maternal history, MAP, UTPI, and serum PlGF. When the risk calculated from this test reaches a certain threshold, patients are classified as high risk and can benefit from interventions. The risk calculator is available free of charge at https://fetalmedicine.org/research/assess/preeclampsia.[24]

Pragmatic Approach

Where resources are limited, routine screening for PE by maternal factors and MAP in all pregnancies should be considered. We can keep reserving measurements of PlGF and UTPI for a subgroup of the population which is classified high risk based on history and BP. This is done

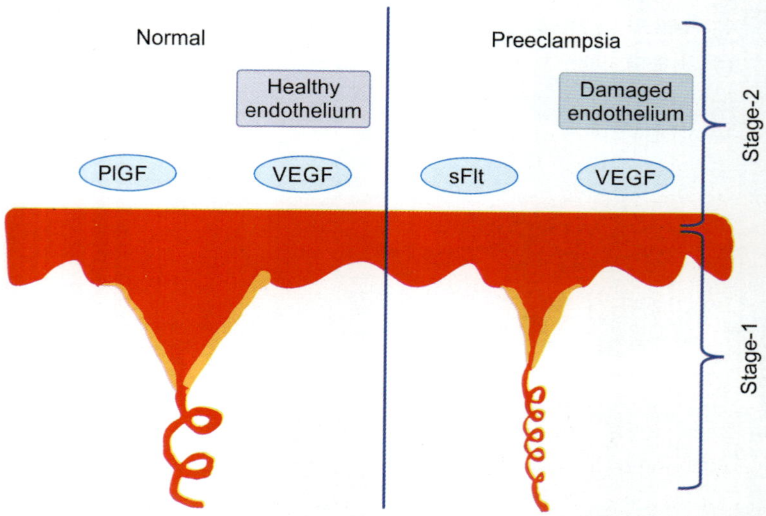

Fig. 2: Pathogenesis of preeclamspsia (stagewise). (PlGF: placental growth factor; sFlt: soluble fms-like tyrosine kinase; VEGF: vascular endothelial growth factor)

because most developing countries around the world are unable to implement a first-trimester screening program for preterm PE based on the combined test because of cost factors. Hence, a practical approach of using history and BP alone is advocated because it can be implemented at a larger scale in low- and middle-income countries and thus can be of great value. Overall sensitivity gets reduced, but the whole approach becomes economically feasible.[25]

Gestosis Score: A Low Resource Setting Tool

A careful history taken early in first trimester can warrant attention for effective prediction and prevention toward mothers "at risk" very early. This can be done by any healthcare worker by using hypertensive disorder of pregnancy-gestosis score. It is an effective and feasible prediction policy.

Process of risk scoring: This score involves all the existing and emerging risk factors in the pregnant woman. Score 1, 2, and 3 is allotted to each clinical risk factor as per its severity in development of PE **(Table 2)**. With careful history and assessment of woman, a total score is obtained time to time. When total score is ≥3, pregnant woman should be marked as "at risk for PE" **(Table 3)** and started on aspirin.[26]

TABLE 2: Risk factor score.

Risk factor	*Score*
Age older than 35 years	1
Age younger than 19 years	1
Maternal anemia	1
Obesity (BMI >30 kg/m^2)	1
Primigravida	1
Short duration of sperm exposure (cohabitation)	1
Woman born as small for gestational age	1
Family history of cardiovascular disease	1
Polycystic ovary syndrome	1
Inter pregnancy interval more than 7 years	1
Conceived with assisted reproductive (IVF/ICSI) treatment	1
MAP >85 mm Hg	1
Chronic vascular disease (dyslipidemia)	1
Excessive weight gain during pregnancy	1
Maternal hypothyroidism	2
Family history of preeclampsia	2
Gestational diabetes mellitus	2
Obesity (BMI >35 kg/m^2)	2
Multifetal pregnancy	2
Hypertensive disease during previous pregnancy	2
Pregestational diabetes mellitus	3
Chronic hypertension	3
Mental disorders	3
Inherited/acquired thrombophilia	3
Maternal chronic kidney disease	3
Autoimmune disease (SLE/APLAS/RA)	3
Pregnancy with assisted reproductive (ovum donation or surrogacy) treatment	3

(BMI: body mass index; IVF/ICSI: in vitro fertilization/intracytoplasmic sperm injection; MAP: mean arterial pressure; SLE/APLAS/RA: systemic lupus erythematosus/antiphospholipid syndrome/rheumatoid arthritis)

DIAGNOSIS AND PREDICTION OF PREECLAMSIA IN LATER GESTATION

Second Trimester

Screening during the 22nd week of gestation is crucial for identifying high-risk individuals for early PE. Combining maternal factors with uterine artery Doppler measurements and PlGF levels significantly enhance the DR.

TABLE 3: Suggested sFlt-1/PlGF ratio cutoffs.[33]

Intention	*Gestation*	*Decision rule*	*sFlt-1/PlGF ratio*
Diagnosis of PE	20–33 + 6 weeks	Rule out cutoff	33
Diagnosis of PE	20–33 + 6 weeks	Rule in cutoff	85
Diagnosis of PE	34 weeks till birth	Rule out cutoff	33
Diagnosis of PE	34 weeks till birth	Rule in cutoff	110
Short-term prediction of PE	24–36 + 6 weeks	Rule out PE for 1 week	38 or less
Short-term prediction of PE	24–36 + 6 weeks	Rule in PE within 4 weeks	Over 38

(PE: preeclampsia; PlGF: placental growth factor; sFlt-1: soluble fms-like tyrosine kinase-1)

Addition of sFlt did not improve sensitivity. This can help in identifying and flagging high-risk patients who would require close monitoring for development of PE.[27]

Screening in Third Trimester

The aim of third-trimester screening is to identify cases of severe PE that may require delivery within 1–4 weeks. Incorporating maternal factors, MAP, UTPI, PlGF, and soluble fms-like tyrosine kinase-1 measurements between 30 and 34 weeks improve sensitivity for prediction of PE. This way, we can closely monitor these pregnancies by frequent BP measurements, proteinuria, and intensive fetal monitoring for growth restriction. Combined screening by maternal factors, MAP, UTPI, PlGF, and sFlt predicted 98% of preterm PE and 49% of term PE at a FPR of 5%.[28,29]

Maternal Ophthalmic Artery

The ophthalmic artery is the first branch of the internal carotid artery and is an easily accessible vessel for Doppler assessment that provides information on the less accessible intracranial circulation. Ophthalmic artery Doppler is a tool that has been studied as an aid in the diagnosis of PE, since its pathogenesis is not limited to the placental bed but extends to cardiovascular and endothelial adaptations during pregnancy.[30] In the 1990s, cross-sectional studies reported that in women with PE, compared with normotensive pregnant women, there is a decrease in impedance to flow and an increase in velocities in the flow velocity waveforms from the ophthalmic arteries. Several studies have described changes in the velocity wave pattern of the ophthalmic artery in women with PE, compared with normotensive pregnant women. In recent prospective observational studies, it was found that the second to first PSV ratio was the ophthalmic artery index that provided useful prediction of PE; the PSV ratio was increased in PE pregnancies and the deviation from normal was greater for earlier PE than later PE.[31,32]

Contingent Screening Model for Screening

Contingent screening model for screening is shown in **Flowchart 1**.

PREDICTION OF PREECLAMPSIA

Prediction of PE is done in women who are at high risk of developing PE. It is done by various methods. Use of markers in the diagnosis of PE:

- *PlGF and sFlt-1/PlGF ratio:* Commercial assays measuring PlGF and sFlt-1/PlGF ratio are recommended for ruling in

Flowchart 1: Contingent screening model.

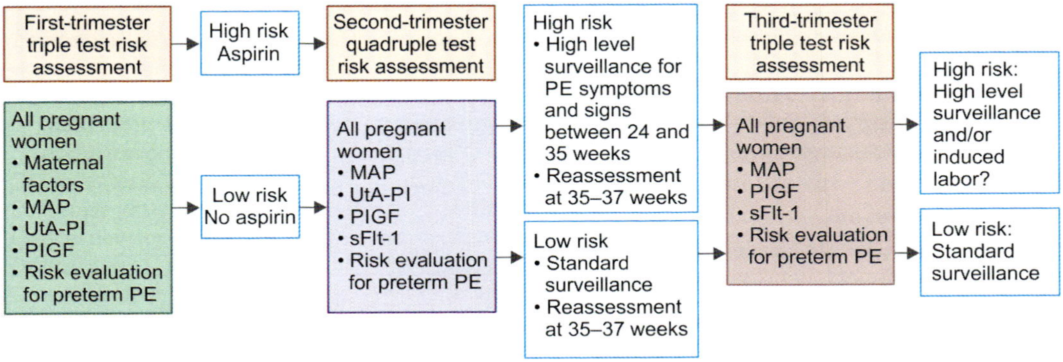

(MAP: mean arterial pressure; PE: preeclampsia; PlGF: placental growth factor; sFlt-1: soluble fms-like tyrosine kinase-1; UtA-PI: uterine artery pulsatility index)

or ruling out PE between 20 and 36 + 6 weeks of gestation. These tests help triage women suspected of having PE based on their clinical symptoms. We should rely on natural clinical pictures rather than only on marker.

- *Congo red urine test:* The Congo red test was initially introduced by Buhimschi et al. This test was used to detect misfolded proteins in the urine of women suspected to have PE. Misfolded proteins have a high binding affinity for Congo red dye.[34] At PE signs and symptoms, the DR was 93% and the FPR 4%. However, with first-trimester urine samples, the DR was 33.3%, 16.1%, and 20% for early, late, and all PE cases, respectively, at 12.8% FPR.[35]
- *Lumella [glycosylated fibronectin (GlyFn)]:* GlyFn point of care test has been validated in a low/middle-income country setting for PE diagnosis and may be a useful adjunctive tool for early identification, appropriate triage, and improved outcomes.[36] Increased levels of GlyFn were seen as of sFlt-1. Sensitivity reported was higher than that of PAPP-A, sFlt-1, and PlGF.[36]

REFERENCES

1. Cunningham FG, Roberts JM, Lindheimer MD (Eds). The clinical spectrum of pre-eclampsia. Chesley's Hypertensive Disorders in Pregnancy, 3rd edition. San Diego, CA: Elsevier; 2009. pp. 25-35.
2. Mol BWJ, Roberts CT, Thangaratinam S, Magee LA, de Groot CJM, Hofmeyr GJ. Preeclampsia. Lancet. 2016;387:999-1011.
3. Duley L. The global impact of preeclampsia and eclampsia. Semin Perinatol. 2009;33:130-7.
4. Kuklina EV, Ayala C, Callaghan WM. Hypertensive disorders and severe obstetric morbidity in the United States. Obstet Gynecol. 2009;113:1299-306.
5. Ackerman CM, Platner MH, Spatz ES, Illuzzi JL, Xu X, Campbell KH, et al. Severe cardiovascular morbidity in women with hypertensive diseases during delivery hospitalization. Am J Obstet Gynecol. 2019;220:582.e1-11.
6. Stevens W, Shih T, Incerti D, Ton TGN, Lee HC, Peneva D, et al. Short term costs of preeclampsia to the United States health care system. Am J Obstet Gynecol. 2017;217:237-48.e16.
7. Hitti J, Sienas L, Walker S, Benedetti TJ, Easterling T. Contribution of hypertension to severe maternal morbidity. Am J Obstet Gynecol. 2018;219:405.e1-7.

8. Carr DB, Newton KM, Utzschneider KM, Tong J, Gerchman F, Kahn SE, et al. Preeclampsia and risk of developing subsequent diabetes. Hypertens Preg. 2009;28:435-47.
9. Magnussen EB, Vatten LJ, Smith GD, Romundstad PR. Hypertensive disorders in pregnancy and subsequently measured cardiovascular risk factors. Obstet Gynecol. 2009;114:961-70.
10. McDonald SD, Han Z, Walsh MW, Gerstein HC, Devereaux PJ. Kidney disease after preeclampsia: a systematic review and meta-analysis. Am J Kidney Dis. 2010;55:1026-39.
11. Witlin GA, Saade GR, Mattar FM, Sibai BM. Predictors of neonatal outcome in women with severe preeclampsia or eclampsia between 24 and 33 week's gestation. Am J Obstet Gynecol. 2000;182:607-11.
12. Tranquilli AL, Brown MA, Zeeman GG, Dekker G, Sibai BM. The definition of severe and early-onset preeclampsia. Statements from the International Society for the Study of Hypertension in Pregnancy (ISSHP). Pregnancy Hypertens. 2013;3:44-7.
13. Roberge S, Villa P, Nicolaides K, Giguere Y, Vainio M, Bakthi A, et al. Early administration of low-dose aspirin for the prevention of preterm and term preeclampsia. A systematic review and meta-analysis. Fetal Diagn Ther. 2012;31:141-6.
14. Roberge S, Nicolaides KH, Demers S, Villa P, Bujold E. Prevention of perinatal death and adverse perinatal outcome using low-dose aspirin: a meta-analysis. Ultrasound Obstet Gynecol. 2013;41:491-9.
15. Rolnik DL, Wright D, Poon LCY, Syngelaki A, O'Gorman N, de Paco Matallana C, et al. ASPRE trial: performance of screening for preterm pre-eclampsia. Ultrasound Obstet Gynecol. 2017;50(4):492-5.
16. Poon LC, Kametas NA, Chelemen T, Leal A, Nicolaides KH. Maternal risk factors for hypertensive disorders in pregnancy: a multivariate approach. J Hum Hypertens. 2010;24:104-10.
17. Committee opinion No. 638: First-trimester risk assessment for early-onset preeclampsia. Obstet Gynecol. 2015;126:e25-27.
18. Tan MY, Syngelaki A, Poon LC, Rolnik DL, O'Gorman N, Delgado JL, et al. Screening for pre-eclampsia by maternal factors and biomarkers at 11–13 weeks' gestation. Ultrasound Obstet Gynecol. 2018;52:186-95.
19. Meekins JW, Pijnenborg R, Hanssens M, McFadyen IR, van Asshe A. A study of placental bed spiral arteries and trophoblastic invasion in normal and severe preeclamptic pregnancies. BJOG. 1994;101: 669-74.
20. Granger JP, Alexander BT, Llinas MT, Bennett WA, Khalil RA. Pathophysiology of hypertension during preeclampsia linking placental ischemia with endothelial dysfunction. Hypertension. 2001;38:718-22.
21. Gallo D, Poon LC, Fernandez M, Wright D, Nicolaides KH. Prediction of preeclampsia by mean arterial pressure at 11–13 and 20–24 week's gestation. Fetal Diagn Ther. 2014;36(1):28-37.
22. Plasencia W, Maiz N, Bonino S, Kaihura C, Nicolaides KH. Uterine artery Doppler at 11 + 0 to 13 + 6 weeks in the prediction of pre-eclampsia. Ultrasound Obstet Gynecol. 2007;30:742-9.
23. Wright D, Syngelaki A, Bradbury I, Akolekar R, Nicolaides KH. First-trimester screening for trisomies 21, 18 and 13 by ultrasound and biochemical testing. Fetal Diagn Ther. 2014;35:118-26.
24. The Fetal Medicine Foundation. Risk assessment. [online] Available from https://fetalmedicine.org/research/assess/preeclampsia/first-trimester [Last accessed March, 2024].
25. Poon LC, Shennan A, Hyett JA, Kapur A, Hadar E, Divakar H, et al. The International Federation of Gynecology and Obstetrics (FIGO) initiative on pre-eclampsia: a pragmatic guide for first-trimester screening and prevention. Int J Gynaecol Obstet. 2019;145(Suppl 1):1-33.
26. FOGSI-GESTOSIS-ICOG. (2019). Hypertensive Disorders in Pregnancy (HDP): Good Clinical Practice Recommendations 2019. [online] Available from https://www.fogsi.org/wp-content/uploads/gcpr/

hdp-fogsi-gestosis-icog-gcpr-2019.pdf [Last accessed March, 2024].
27. Gallo DM, Wright D, Casanova C, Campanero M, Nicolaides KH. Competing risks model in screening for preeclampsia by maternal factors and biomarkers at 19–24 weeks' gestation. Am J Obstet Gynecol. 2016;214: 619.e1-17.
28. Tsiakkas A, Saiid Y, Wright A, Wright D, Nicolaides KH. Competing risks model in screening for preeclampsia by maternal factors and biomarkers at 30–34 weeks' gestation. Am J Obstet Gynecol. 2016;215(1):87.
29. Zeisler H, Llurba E, Chantraine F, Vatish M, Staff AC, Sennström M, et al. Predictive value of the sFlt-1: PlGF ratio in women with suspected preeclampsia. N Engl J Med. 2016;374:13.
30. Gurgel Alves JA, Praciano de Sousa PC, Bezerra Maia E Holanda Moura S, Kane SC, da Silva Costa F. First-trimester maternal ophthalmic artery Doppler analysis for prediction of pre-eclampsia. Ultrasound Obstet Gynecol. 2014;44:411-8.
31. Matias DS, Costa RF, Matias BS, Gordiano L, Correia LC. Predictive value of ophthalmic artery Doppler velocimetry in relation to development of pre-eclampsia. Ultrasound Obstet Gynecol. 2014;44:419-26.
32. Praciano de Souza PC, Gurgel Alves JA, Bezerra Maia E Holanda Moura S, Araujo Júnior E, Martins WP, Da Silva Costa F. Second trimester screening of preeclampsia using maternal characteristics and uterine and ophthalmic artery Doppler. Ultraschall Med. 2018;39:190-7.
33. National Institute for Clinical Excellence. (2022). PLGF-based testing to help diagnose suspected preterm pre-eclampsia: Diagnostics Guidance. [online] Available from http://www.nice.org.uk/guidance/dg49 [Last accessed March, 2024].
34. Khaliq OP, Phoswa WN, Moodley J. The effectiveness of the Congo Red Dot paper test in hypertensive disorders of pregnancy: A systematic review and meta-analysis. Front Reprod Health. 2023;5:1120937.
35. Sammar M, Syngelaki A, Sharabi-Nov A, Nicolaides K, Meiri H. Can Staining of Damaged Proteins in Urine Effectively Predict Preeclampsia? Fetal Diagn Ther. 2017;41(1):23-31.
36. Nagalla SR, Janaki V, Vijayalakshmi AR, Chayadevi K, Pratibha D, Rao PV, et al. Glycosylated fibronectin point-of-care test for diagnosis of pre-eclampsia in a low-resource setting: a prospective Southeast Asian population study. BJOG. 2020;127(13): 1687-94.

4

CHAPTER

Knobology: Optimizing the Image

Alok Varshney

KEY POINTS

1. Optimizing ultrasound images is essential for obtaining accurate diagnostic information and enhancing the quality of patient care.
2. It is important to consider the specific clinical requirements, patient factors, and operator expertise when applying these optimization strategies.
3. Image quality primarily depends on the ultrasound probe's frequency, but higher frequencies also increase attenuation, limiting the depth of view.
4. Position the area of interest as close as possible to the probe.
5. Optimize the scan area by adjusting depth, sector width, and zoom.
6. Brightness and contrast can be improved by adjusting gain, time gain compensation (TGC), and dynamic contrast settings.
7. Modern techniques such as tissue harmonic imaging and compound imaging enhance image quality, while postprocessing methods such as speckle reduction and the application of various grayscale and color maps can further enhance the images.

INTRODUCTION

Ultrasound knobology refers to the understanding and operation of the various knobs and controls on an ultrasound machine.[1] These controls are used to adjust the imaging parameters and optimize the ultrasound image quality for different types of examinations and patient conditions.

BASIC PHYSICS

Understanding ultrasound physics is essential for the proper operation and interpretation of ultrasound imaging equipment.[2] Some key concepts are outlined further:

- *Sound:* It is the transmission of pressure waves through a medium, wherein each wave cycle consists of a complete positive and negative pressure shift **(Fig. 1)**. The *wavelength* denotes the distance covered during a single cycle. The *frequency* of the wave is measured in Hertz (cycles/s, Hz), representing the number of cycles per second. *Amplitude* describes the strength of a wave, which determines the loudness or intensity of sound.[3]
- *Ultrasound waves:* They are high-frequency sound waves with frequencies above the upper limit of human hearing (typically, >20,000 Hz). In diagnostic ultrasound, frequencies between 2 and 20 million Hertz (Megahertz: MHz) are commonly used.[3] These waves propagate through tissues and are used to create detailed images of the body's internal structures.
- *Attenuation:* Attenuation refers to the gradual weakening of ultrasound waves as they travel through tissues. Factors such

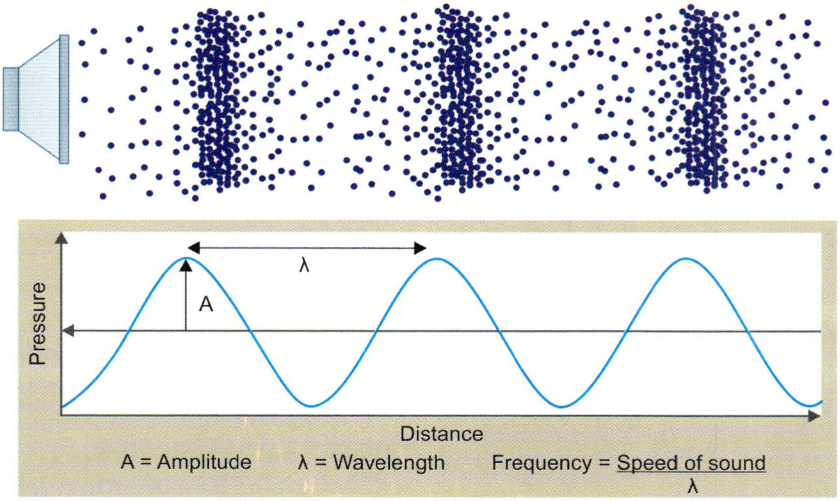

Fig. 1: A sound wave that induces compression and rarefaction within a medium. The wave's crests represent high-pressure regions, while the troughs represent low-pressure regions.

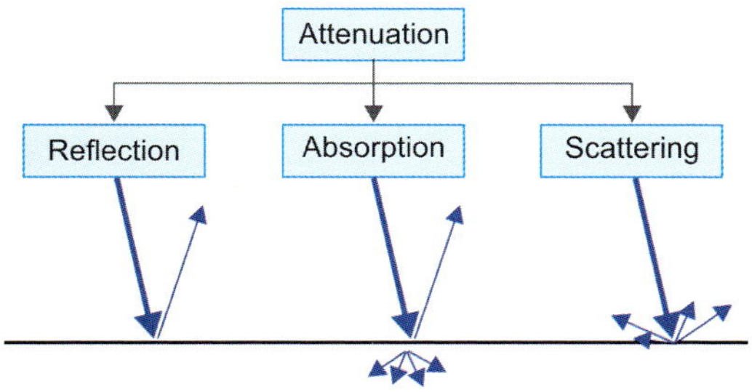

Fig. 2: Attenuation of a sound wave as it encounters an interface. The wave can undergo reflection, absorption, and scattering processes.

as reflection, absorption, and scattering contribute to attenuation **(Fig. 2)**. Attenuation is frequency dependent, with higher frequencies experiencing greater attenuation than lower frequencies.[4]

- *Reflection:* When ultrasound waves encounter a boundary between two tissues with different acoustic properties, such as density or stiffness, a portion of the wave is reflected toward the transducer. The reflected waves create the echoes used to form the ultrasound image.[5]
- *Absorption:* It occurs when ultrasound waves are converted into heat energy as they pass through tissues. Tissues with higher absorption properties, such as bones, attenuate ultrasound waves more than tissues with lower absorption.[4]
- *Scattering:* It refers to the random redirection of ultrasound waves by small structures within tissues. Scattering contributes to the overall "speckle" pattern seen in ultrasound images and can affect image quality.[6]

IMAGE GENERATION

Ultrasound imaging involves using high-frequency sound waves to create images of the body's internal structures. The key components for image generation are:

- *Transducers:* Ultrasound imaging relies on transducers, which are devices that convert electrical energy into ultrasound waves and vice versa. Transducers contain *piezoelectric crystals* that generate sound waves when an electrical current is applied to them and produce electrical signals when sound waves strike them.[2,7]

Crystals are arranged along a curved (convex) surface in *convex transducers* (curved linear array) **(Fig. 3A)**. This enables a wide field of view and good depth of display. *Linear transducers* (linear array) use crystals arranged in a straight line, generating ultrasound waves in parallel and producing a higher and more uniform resolution **(Fig. 3B)**.[7] However, they have limited depth penetration as high frequencies are used. *Intracavity transducers* are used for transvaginal or transrectal sonography. These have crystals arranged at the tip of a long and slim probe **(Fig. 3C)**. In most machines, it is possible to select the appropriate probe for a study by simply pressing a button or touching the probe icon on a screen.

- *Pulse-echo method:* This method is the basis of ultrasound imaging.[3] An ultrasound transducer emits short pulses of ultrasound waves, which then travel through the tissues. When these waves encounter boundaries between different tissues or organs, they are reflected back as echoes to the transducer. The transducer detects these echoes and converts them into electrical signals. The signals are processed in the form of *scan lines*, which are individual lines of data acquired by the transducer. Sequential scan lines are combined to generate a two-dimensional (2D) image on the ultrasound screen **(Figs. 4A and B)**. By continuously transmitting and receiving pulses of sound waves and combining the scan lines, real-time ultrasound imaging is achieved.[2,7]

ULTRASOUND IMAGING MODES

During the scan, real-time images of the tissue anatomy and motion can be obtained in *B-mode* (brightness mode) and *M-mode* (motion mode). *Color Doppler, continuous-wave,* and *pulse-wave Doppler* combine B-mode imaging with the Doppler effect. *Three-dimensional (3D) ultrasound* uses specialized probes and advanced software to capture multiple 2D images from different angles, combining them to form a 3D volume image. This volume image provides a more detailed and realistic representation of the anatomical structures being imaged. *Four-dimensional (4D) ultrasound* builds upon 3D ultrasound by adding the element of time, creating a real-time video or live-motion view of the 3D volume, which is useful for assessing fetal movements, facial expressions, or capturing dynamic events.

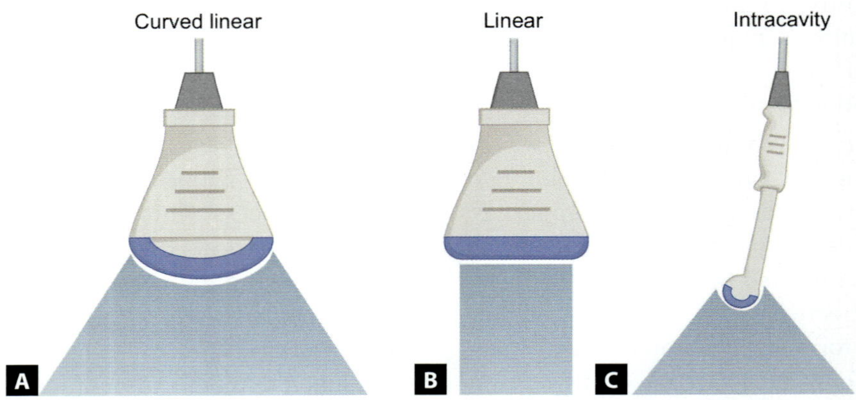

Figs. 3A to C: Commonly used transducers or probes in obstetric ultrasound examinations.

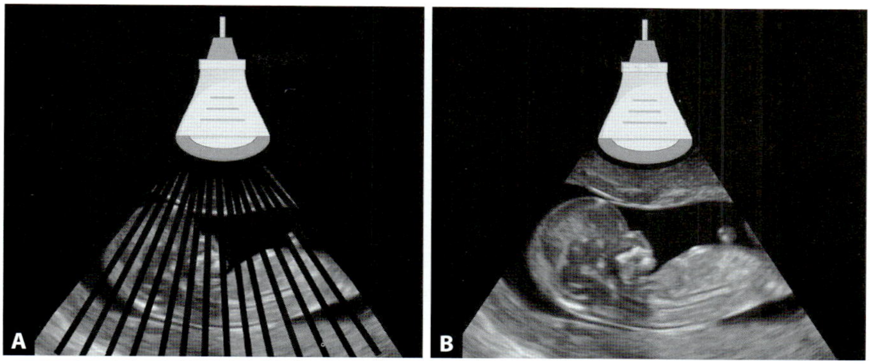

Figs. 4A and B: Illustration of scan lines. These refer to the individual lines or beams of ultrasound waves that are transmitted and received during the imaging process. Each scan line represents a single beam of ultrasound that is transmitted and received at a specific angle, typically in a sweeping motion. By combining multiple scan lines at different angles, an image of the internal structures of the body is created.

BIOEFFECTS AND SAFETY CONSIDERATIONS

Sound waves are a form of energy that have the potential to cause effects on tissues.[8] The measure of the energy of the ultrasound beams is called *acoustic power*. The parameters that determine the acoustic power are:

- *Power:* Total amount of energy delivered by the ultrasound system per unit of time is called power. It is typically expressed in units of watts (W). Higher power levels can result in increased signal strength and penetration but should be carefully controlled to ensure patient safety.[8]
- *Intensity:* Ultrasound intensity refers to the power per unit area of the ultrasound beam. It is typically expressed in units of watts per square centimeter (W/cm^2). The intensity of the ultrasound beam can vary depending on factors such as the system settings, transducer characteristics, and imaging mode.[9,10]
- *Mechanical index (MI):* It is a parameter that indicates the potential for bioeffects related to the mechanical actions of ultrasound waves. It represents the ratio of the peak negative pressure to the square root of the ultrasound frequency. The MI is used to assess the likelihood of cavitation (formation of gas bubbles) and other mechanical effects. Lower MI values indicate lower risk, while higher values suggest higher potential for mechanical effects.[10,11]
- *Thermal index (TI):* It is a parameter that quantifies the potential for tissue heating due to ultrasound exposure. It is expressed as a ratio and is dependent on factors such as the power, duration, and frequency of the ultrasound waves. Higher TI values indicate a higher potential for heating effects. Multiple TI values may be provided for different tissue types to account for variations in thermal sensitivity.[11]
- *Safety guidelines:* Healthcare professionals operating ultrasound systems should adhere to safety guidelines to ensure that the acoustic output remains within acceptable limits for the safe and effective use of ultrasound for diagnostic purposes. The guiding principle is "ALARA", which stands for "as low as reasonably achievable" acoustic power.[7,9] Regulatory bodies, such as the Food and

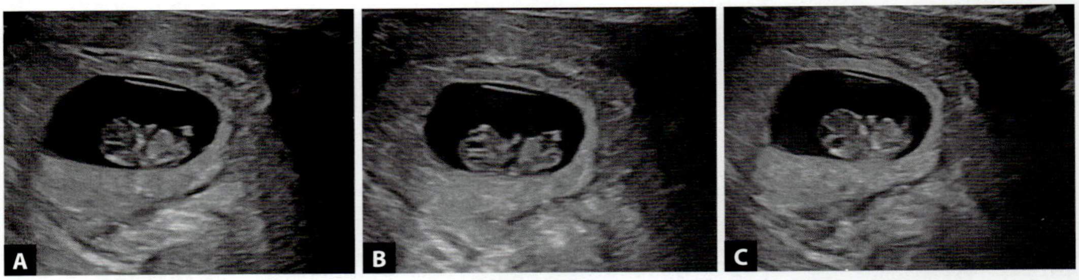

Figs. 5A to C: Comparative images captured during a first-trimester scan, showcasing the impact of different acoustic power (AP) and gain settings on the mechanical index (MI): (A) AP 95% (MI 1.0); (B) AP 70% (MI 0.5); (C) AP 50% (MI 0.3).

Note: Lowering the acoustic power while increasing the gain yields a high-quality image while maintaining a lower mechanical index.

Drug Administration (FDA) in the United States, provide guidelines on maximum allowable acoustic output levels for different applications.[12]

Tip: High acoustic power should be avoided while doing fetal ultrasound to minimize bioeffects. Good-quality ultrasound images can be generated by adjusting the overall gain and reducing the acoustic power **(Figs. 5A to C)**.

RESOLUTION OF AN IMAGE

The resolution is a measure of the level of detail or clarity that can be achieved in the ultrasound image for an accurate representation of the body part being examined. There are three types of resolutions in ultrasound imaging:[7]

1. *Spatial resolution:* It refers to the ability to distinguish small structures that are close together. It determines the level of detail in the image. Spatial resolution is typically described in terms of axial resolution and lateral resolution.[4]
   a. Axial resolution: It is also known as depth resolution, which refers to the ability to distinguish structures along the depth or axial direction of the ultrasound beam. It is determined by the frequency and duration of the ultrasound waves (pulse length).[4] A higher frequency and a shorter pulse length result in better axial resolution.[7]
   b. *Lateral resolution:* It is also called transverse resolution, which refers to the ability to distinguish structures perpendicular to the ultrasound beam. It is influenced by factors such as the width of the ultrasound beam, focusing techniques, and the frequency of the ultrasound waves. A narrower beam and higher frequency contribute to better lateral resolution.[4,5]
2. *Temporal resolution:* It is a measure of how well the ultrasound system can track and represent dynamic movements or events in real time. It is typically described in terms of *frame rate*, which represents the number of image frames displayed per second (fps).[7] A higher frame rate provides better temporal resolution, allowing for a smoother and more accurate representation of dynamic events.[2,7] For example, in fetal cardiac imaging, a higher frame rate is necessary to visualize the fast movements of the structures of the heart.
3. *Contrast resolution:* It refers to the ability to differentiate between subtle differences in tissue echogenicity or grayscale variations in the ultrasound image.

Contrast resolution is influenced by factors such as the image gain settings, the dynamic range of the ultrasound system, and the underlying tissue characteristics.[2,7]

Spatial resolution, temporal resolution, and contrast resolution are crucial for the accurate diagnosis and interpretation of ultrasound images. The optimal balance of these depends on the specific imaging requirements, clinical applications, and the characteristics of the structures or pathologies being imaged.[2,4]

OPTIMIZING IMAGE ACQUISITION

To ensure the acquisition of a high-quality image, the way we acquire the image plays a crucial role. The guiding principle for achieving optimal image acquisition involves positioning the area of interest as close as possible to the ultrasound probe. When the area being examined is situated farther away, the ultrasound beam experiences greater attenuation, resulting in degraded image quality.[3] Several techniques can be employed to acquire optimum images, including:

- *Utilizing thin sections of the maternal abdomen:* Thin areas of the maternal abdomen, such as the suprapubic region, umbilicus, and flanks, offer favorable acoustic windows for imaging the fetus. Locating a suitable acoustic window becomes particularly important in patients with a high body mass index (BMI).[13]
- *Applying probe pressure:* Gentle pressure applied to the maternal abdomen using the probe can effectively bring the fetal part under examination closer to the probe, thus improving the resolution of the image.
- *Transvaginal sonography (TVS):* It employs high-frequency transducers to generate images. Moreover, the fetal part being examined is close to the TVS probe, minimizing attenuation.[13] TVS is frequently utilized to produce images with an excellent resolution during the first trimester and in specialized examinations like fetal neurosonography.

IMAGE OPTIMIZATION

Optimizing the Scan Area

- *Depth adjustment:* The depth knob on the ultrasound machine allows for vertical sizing of the imaging window, enabling visualization of structures at different depths within the body. Altering this setting helps in examining superficial or deeper organs as required. The depth setting is influenced by factors such as transducer frequency, transmission power, and tissue harmonic imaging (THI).[7,14] Increasing the depth setting leads to slower image acquisition and reduced frame rate due to the longer travel time of the echo signal from deeper structures. Additionally, higher depths result in greater attenuation of the sound beam, leading to decreased image resolution.[15] Moreover, increasing the depth setting introduces more noise into the image, as the ultrasound system finds it challenging to distinguish genuine ultrasonic signals from background noise artifacts.[7] Consequently, reducing the depth setting enhances image quality **(Figs. 6A and B)**.

  Tip: To begin the examination, it is advisable to use a high-depth setting to obtain an orientation and overall view of the anatomy. Once the structures of interest have been identified, the depth should be decreased to minimize the display of irrelevant deeper structures.

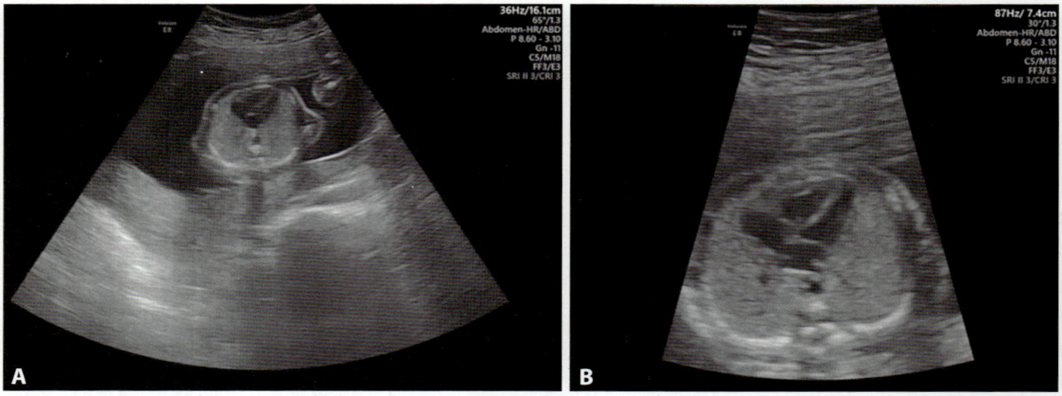

Figs. 6A and B: Comparative images obtained during a fetal heart examination, demonstrating the influence of modifying depth and sector width settings on the frame rate: (A) With a high depth and a wide sector width, the resulting frame rate is 36 Hz; (B) By reducing the depth and narrowing the sector width to exclude irrelevant areas from the scanning field, a high-quality image with a significantly improved frame rate of 87 Hz can be achieved, enhancing the temporal resolution.

- *Sector width adjustment:* The sector width knob is used to modify the width of the image when using a sector probe. Reducing the sector width decreases the number of scan lines and reduces the computational requirements for image creation, resulting in improved resolution and frame rate.[5] Adjusting the sector width is particularly important when evaluating moving structures, such as the fetal heart **(Figs. 6A and B)**.

  Tip: To begin the examination, use a wide sector width to obtain an overall view of the anatomy. Then, gradually reduce the width to encompass only the structures of interest.
- *Zoom function:* The zoom feature allows for magnification of a specific area within the ultrasound image, facilitating detailed examination of structures and finer details. There are two types of zoom functions available. "Read zoom" involves digitally magnifying a frozen image, while "write zoom" enables zooming in on a section of the live image during scanning.[2,7,15] When utilizing write zoom, the echoes outside the remaining scan area are no longer evaluated, which increases the line density in the zoomed area, thereby improving temporal resolution. On the other hand, read zoom does not enhance image resolution.[1,7]

  Tip: Whenever possible, utilize write zoom to avoid compromising image resolution.

Optimizing Image Brightness and Contrast

- *Overall gain adjustment:* The overall gain knob is used to control the brightness of the ultrasound image by amplifying or reducing the strength of the echo signals returning from the body. Increasing the gain enhances weak echoes, making them more visible and improving contrast resolution. However, excessive gain can lead to an overly bright image. On the other hand, reducing the gain can help reduce excessive brightness caused by strong echoes but may result in a darker image **(Figs. 7A to C)**. The overall gain allows for the improvement of image

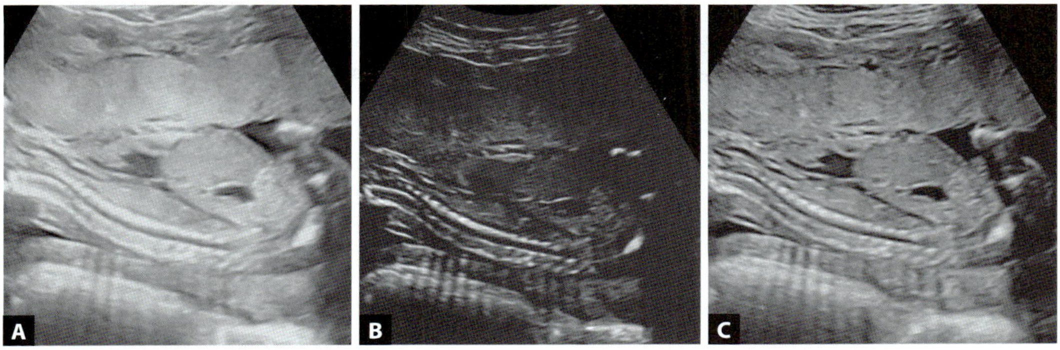

Figs. 7A to C: Comparative images acquired during a fetal examination, highlighting the impact of adjusting the overall gain settings on image quality: (A) Image obtained with a high gain setting, resulting in excessive brightness and the presence of echoes in typically echo-free regions; (B) Image obtained with a low gain setting, resulting in a darker image; (C) By optimizing the gain adjustment, a high-quality image can be obtained, accurately representing the varying echo intensities of different tissues.

quality by adjusting the brightness of the entire field of view without increasing the intensity of the transmitted sound energy.[1,2,7]

Tip: Adjust the gain in a way that echoes should not be visible in structures that are typically echo-free, such as the urinary bladder or gallbladder.

- *Time gain compensation adjustment:* The TGC knobs enable fine-tuning of the echo signals at specific depths. This compensation is necessary to account for the attenuation or weakening of sound waves as they travel deeper into the body. By adjusting the TGC controls, more uniform brightness can be achieved throughout the image, compensating for variations in tissue attenuation.[1,5,7]

  Tip: At the beginning of the examination, center all the TGC settings. After adjusting the overall gain, fine-tune the TGC to compensate for attenuation at specific depths, ensuring a consistent image brightness.
- *Dynamic range adjustment:* The dynamic range control on the ultrasound system enables the operator to specify the range of gray shades to be displayed on the monitor. A high dynamic range corresponds to a greater number of gray shades assigned for displaying echo intensities, resulting in a smoother image. Conversely, a low dynamic range limits the number of available gray shades, leading to higher contrast between regions with different echogenicities.[1,7]

  Tip: The dynamic range serves as the contrast button on the ultrasound machine and can be easily adjusted to achieve softer or high-contrast images according to preference **(Figs. 8A to C)**.

Optimizing Resolution

- *Transducer selection:* The choice of transducer depends on specific clinical requirements, the type of examination being performed, maternal body habitus, and the expertise of the sonographer. The transducer frequency determines the resolution and penetration depth of the ultrasound waves.[6] Higher frequencies (5–12 MHz) offer a superior resolution for evaluating superficial structures and detecting abnormalities in fetal anatomy. Lower frequencies (2–5 MHz) provide greater penetration for visualizing

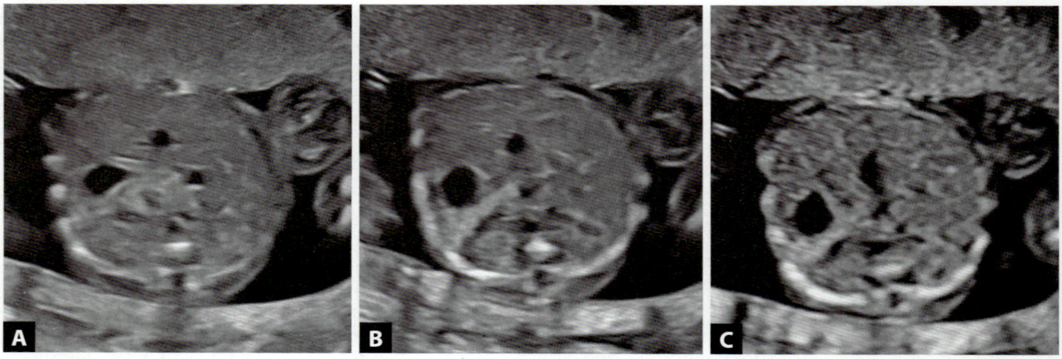

Figs. 8A to C: Comparative images of the fetal abdomen, showcasing the impact of adjusting the dynamic range settings on image contrast: (A) Image obtained with a high dynamic range setting, resulting in a low-contrast image, lacking noticeable contrast between different anatomical structures; (B) Image acquired with a midrange dynamic range setting, providing optimal contrast with clear differentiation between various tissues; (C) Image obtained with a low dynamic range setting, producing a high-contrast image. This can be beneficial in certain scenarios where highlighting specific details or abnormalities is of particular interest.

deeper structures such as the fetal heart or spine but may compromise some resolution.[1,7]

Tip: A high-frequency probe should be used for first- and second-trimester obstetric scans. A low-frequency probe may be needed for scanning in the third trimester or a patient with a high BMI.

- *Focus/focal zone:* The focus control narrows the width of the ultrasound beam at a specific depth using electronic means.[1,2,7] The focal zone can be adjusted up or down by the operator and should be positioned at the region of interest or posterior to it.[15] This adjustment improves spatial resolution at that particular depth. If multiple focal zones are selected by the operator, resolution can be improved at multiple depths. However, increasing the number of focal zones also reduces the frame rate, thereby decreasing temporal resolution.[7]

Other Techniques

- *Tissue harmonic imaging:* In conventional ultrasound imaging, the transducer emits sound waves at a specific frequency and the echoes received from tissues are captured at the same frequency. However, THI exploits the phenomenon in which tissues produce harmonic frequencies that are double the transmitted frequency. The ultrasound system employs advanced signal processing techniques to isolate and capture these harmonic frequencies. As a result, images are obtained with improved penetration and resolution, along with reduced noise, enabling better visualization of structures, especially in near-field regions or deep tissues.[1,2,7]

  Tip: For optimal image quality in fetal imaging, it is recommended to keep harmonic imaging enabled. However, in certain scenarios, such as when evaluating fetal bones, harmonic imaging may be switched off to avoid the smoothening effect it can produce.
- *Compound imaging:* In traditional ultrasound imaging, a single beam is used to capture an image in a straight line. However, compound imaging employs the generation of multiple beams at

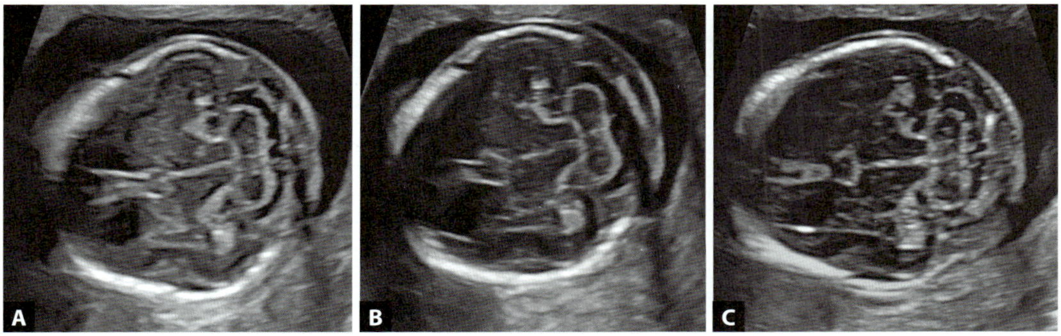

Figs. 9A to C: Comparative visualization of a fetal head using various gray maps. The images remain unaltered in all other aspects. Note the distinct contrast variations depicted in the three images.

different angles or frequencies, resulting in multiple ultrasound images obtained from various perspectives. These images are then combined to create a composite image that exhibits improved clarity and reduced artifacts. Compound imaging offers several advantages, including enhanced edge definition, improved visualization of subtle structures, and a reduction in artifacts such as speckle noise.[7,16] However, it is important to note that compound imaging may impart an overly smooth appearance to the image and may lead to the loss of shadowing artifacts.[17]

Postprocessing

Postprocessing techniques are valuable for further enhancing the quality and perception of ultrasound images.[7,18] These techniques can be applied to both live and stored images.

- *Gray maps:* While the dynamic range determines the total number of gray shades available to represent ultrasound signals, a gray map determines the brightness or darkness of each shade of gray displayed on the screen.[7,19] Modifying the gray map can improve or reduce the perception of image contrast, depending on the examiner's preference **(Figs. 9A to C)**.
- *Chromatic colors:* The gray scale can also be represented using different colors. This approach is based on the understanding that human eyes have higher resolution in color vision compared to black and white.[20] Applying color maps to ultrasound images can enhance image contrast and make them visually appealing **(Figs. 10A to F)**. However, the choice of color mapping is subjective and dependent on the examiner's preference.[7]
- *Speckle reduction:* It is an algorithm-based technique that aims to reduce speckle noise, thereby minimizing the graininess of the image. This can be achieved through techniques such as *spatial averaging* (averaging multiple ultrasound frames or scan lines), *filtering* to suppress high-frequency noise, and *image postprocessing* where brighter pixels are enhanced and darker pixels are suppressed.[21,22] Speckle reduction techniques aim to improve image quality. However, it is important to note that the reduction of noise can result in a smoothening effect, which may lead to a decrease in image resolution, less sharp edges, and loss of fine details.[7]

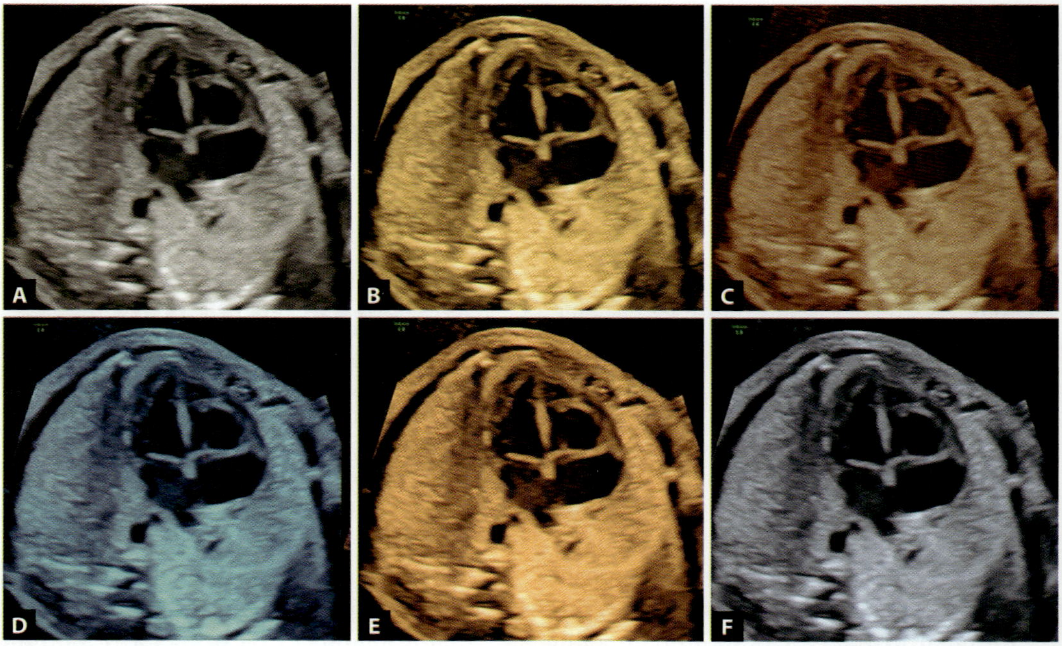

Figs. 10A to F: Application of different color maps to the fetal heart images. Color tints can improve the image contrast and enhance image quality and aesthetic appeal subjectively.

Organizing the Machine Settings

- *Presets:* They are preconfigured settings on an ultrasound machine that are specifically designed to optimize image acquisition for particular types of examinations or anatomical regions.[7,15] These presets serve as standardized starting points, allowing operators to efficiently obtain high-quality images.[5] Each preset is assembled with specific imaging parameters, such as transducer frequency, depth settings, gain, TGC, focal zones, and image processing settings, customized to suit the characteristics of the target anatomy or clinical application.[1] Ultrasound presets can be customized and given names according to the individual operator's specific needs.
- *Auto-optimization:* It is a feature found in many modern ultrasound machines that enables quick and automatic adjustment of imaging parameters to optimize image quality at the touch of a button, eliminating the need for manual adjustments by the operator.[23] This feature utilizes algorithms and advanced image processing techniques to analyze the acquired ultrasound data in real-time, automatically adjusting various parameters to enhance image quality and optimize visualization of anatomical structures.[7] However, while auto-optimization can provide a good initial image quality, manual adjustments may still be necessary in certain cases or for specific imaging requirements.

REFERENCES

1. Amo Wiafe Y, Badu-Peprah A. The Influence of Ultrasound Equipment Knobology in Abdominal Sonography. In: Abdo Gamie SA, Foda EM (Eds). Essentials of Abdominal Ultrasound. London: IntechOpen; 2019.

2. Grogan SP, Mount CA. Ultrasound Physics and Instrumentation. In: StatPearls [Internet]. Treasure Island (FL): StatPearls Publishing; 2023.
3. Au A, Zwank M. (2020). Ultrasound Physics and Technical Facts for the Beginner. [online] Available from https://www.acep.org/sonoguide/basic/ultrasound-physics-and-technical-facts-for-the-beginner [Last accessed March, 2024].
4. Tole NM; WHO/Diagnostic Imaging and Laboratory Technology. Basic physics of ultrasonographic imaging. Geneva, Switzerland: World Health Organization; 2005.
5. Xu D. (2019). Physics of Ultrasound. [online] Available from https://www.nysora.com/topics/equipment/physics-of-ultrasound/ [Last accessed March, 2024].
6. Radiology Key. (2020). Physics of ultrasound. [online] Available from https://radiologykey.com/physics-of-ultrasound-3/ [Last accessed March, 2024].
7. Zander D, Hüske S, Hoffmann B, Cui X-W, Dong Y, Lim A, et al. Ultrasound Image Optimization ("Knobology"): B-Mode. Ultrasound Int Open. 2020;06(01):E14-24.
8. Miller DL. Update on safety of diagnostic ultrasonography. J Clin Ultrasound. 1991;19(9):531-40.
9. Nyborg WL. Biological effects of ultrasound: Development of safety guidelines. Part II: General review. Ultrasound Med Biol. 2001;27(3):301-33.
10. Hershkovitz R, Sheiner E, Mazor M. Ultrasound in obstetrics: a review of safety. Eur J Obstet Gynecol Reprod Biol. 2002;101(1):15-8.
11. Nowicki A. Safety of ultrasonic examinations; thermal and mechanical indices. Med Ultrason. 2020;22(2):203.
12. Nelson TR, Fowlkes JB, Abramowicz JS, Church CC. Ultrasound Biosafety Considerations for the Practicing Sonographer and Sonologist. J Ultrasound Med. 2009;28(2):139-50.
13. Paladini D. Sonography in obese and overweight pregnant women: Clinical, medicolegal and technical issues. Ultrasound Obstet Gynecol. 2009;33(6):720-9.
14. Leibovitz Z, Karayanni R, Degani S, Zreik A, Odeh M, Shapiro I, et al. OP33.01: Effect of harmonic imaging, SRI-II, CRI, FFC and coded excitation B-mode features on fetal bowel echogenicity, studied by computerized image analysis. Ultrasound Obstet Gynecol. 2010;36(S1):147.
15. Enriquez JL, Wu TS. An Introduction to Ultrasound Equipment and Knobology. Crit Care Clin. 2014;30(1):25-45.
16. Contreras Ortiz SH, Chiu T, Fox MD. Ultrasound image enhancement: a review. Biomed Signal Process Control. 2012;7(5):419-28.
17. Hung ALY, Galeotti J. Good and bad boundaries in ultrasound compounding: preserving anatomic boundaries while suppressing artifacts. Int J Comput Assist Radiol Surg. 2021;16(11):1957-68.
18. Perperidis A. Postprocessing Approaches for the Improvement of Cardiac Ultrasound B-Mode Images: A Review. IEEE Trans Ultrason Ferroelectr Freq Control. 2016;63(3):470-85.
19. Hedrick WR, Hykes DL. Image and Signal Processing in Diagnostic Ultrasound Imaging. J Diagn Med Sonogr. 1989;5(5):231-9.
20. Dambrosio F, Amy D, Colombo A. B-mode color sonographic images in obstetrics and gynecology: preliminary report. Ultrasound Obstet Gynecol. 1995;6(3):208-15.
21. Hiremath PS, Akkasaligar PT, Badiger S. Speckle Noise Reduction in Medical Ultrasound Images. In: Gunarathne G (Ed). Advancements and Breakthroughs in Ultrasound Imaging. London: IntechOpen; 2013.
22. Park J, Kang JB, Chang JH, Yoo Y. Speckle reduction techniques in medical ultrasound imaging. Biomed Eng Lett. 2014;4(1):32-40.
23. Barr RG, Grajo JR. Dynamic Automatic Ultrasound Optimization. Ultrasound Q. 2009;25(2):63-5.

CHAPTER 5

Basics of Fetal Biometry and Doppler

Ritika Bajaj

KEY POINTS

1. Ultrasound is a very important tool for assessment of fetal growth and placental function.
2. First-trimester fetal biometry involves measurement of crown rump length (CRL) of fetus which is the most reliable method for dating pregnancy.
3. Routine fetal biometry in second and third trimester involves measurement of biparietal diameter (BPD), head circumference (HC), abdominal circumference (AC), and femur length (FL).
4. Estimated fetal weight can be calculated by different formulas which incorporate varied combinations of fetal BPD, HC, AC, and FL.
5. Longitudinal fetal growth charts help to study fetal growth over multiple visits.
6. Biometry measurements using centiles are easy to understand and cutoff point below 10th centile for gestation for AC and/or estimated fetal weight (EFW) have been incorporated into definitions for fetal growth restriction (FGR).
7. Umbilical artery (UA) Doppler waveform is used to study downstream resistance in placental circulation.
8. In fetal hypoxemia, there is central redistribution of blood flow which is reflected as increase in diastolic flow in middle cerebral artery (MCA) and decrease in its pulsatility index.
9. MCA peak systolic velocity (PSV) >1.5 multiple of the median (MoM) is used as a marker for fetal anemia.
10. Ductus venosus normally has a triphasic waveform. Reversal of flow in ductus venosus (DV) during atrial systole ("a" wave) is seen in cases of cardiac dysfunction or fetal acidemia.
11. Abnormal uterine artery Doppler waveform [increase in pulsatility index (PI), early diastolic notch] is used to predict risk of preeclampsia and FGR.

INTRODUCTION

Accurate measurement of fetal biometry is important to identify fetuses at risk of adverse pregnancy outcome. This includes both small for gestational age (SGA) and large for gestational age (LGA) babies. Fetal biometry assessment also has implications for timing and mode of delivery. Ultrasound, if performed correctly, is the most reliable tool for accurate assessment of fetal biometry throughout pregnancy.

FIRST-TRIMESTER BIOMETRY

First-trimester fetal biometry involves measuring the length of fetus from top of head to bottom of rump, commonly called crown rump length **(Fig. 1)**. For correct measurement of CRL, midsagittal section of fetus should be imaged. Fetus should be horizontal (at 90° to the angle of insonation) and in neutral position, i.e., neither

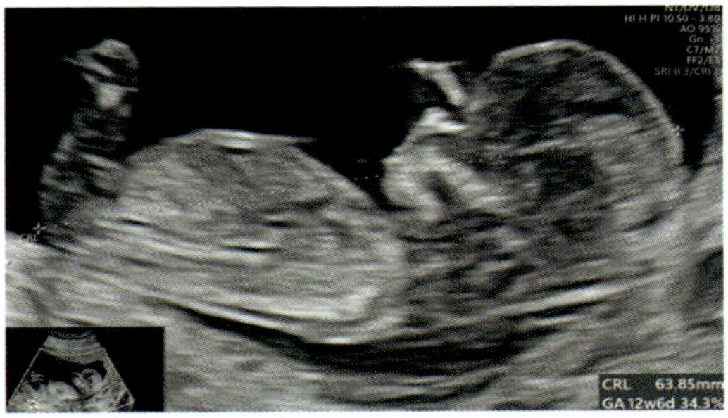

Fig. 1: Crown rump length (CRL) measurement in midsagittal plane of fetus. Both top of head and rump are clearly visible.

hyperextended nor hyperflexed. Image should be appropriately magnified (filling at least 75% of monitor screen). Both the top of head and rump should be clearly visible on ultrasound for accurate placement of calipers. Dating based upon CRL measured between 8 and 14 weeks pregnancy appears to be the most reliable method for dating of pregnancy with a presumed accuracy of ±5 days.[1] Once CRL exceeds 84 mm, head circumference (HC) and/or femur length (FL) should be used for pregnancy dating.

SECOND- AND THIRD-TRIMESTER BIOMETRY

Routine fetal biometry measurement for assessment of fetal weight in second and third trimester incorporates two measurements of fetal head, i.e., biparietal diameter (BPD) and head circumference (HC), one measurement of fetal abdomen, i.e., abdominal circumference (AC) and one measurement of fetal femur, i.e., femur length (FL).

HEAD MEASUREMENTS

Step 1: Obtaining Image

Fetal head measurements (BPD and HC) can be assessed in the transthalamic (TT) plane or transventricular (TV) plane. While biometry in TV plane may yield a slightly

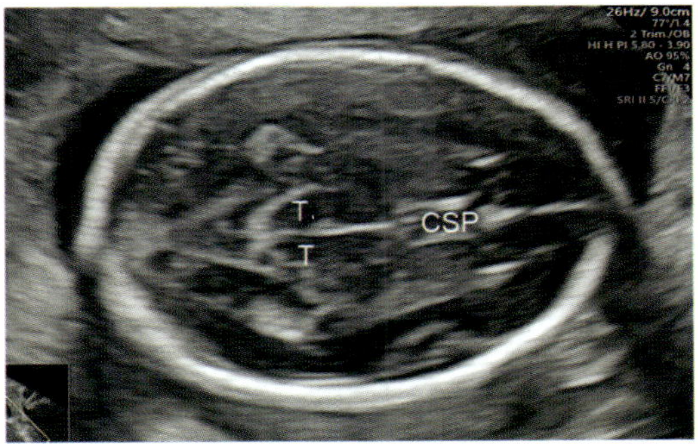

Fig. 2: Transthalamic plane of fetal head used to measure BPD and HC. Falx cerebri, CSP, and paired thalami can be seen. (BPD: biparietal diameter; CSP: cavum septum pellucidum; HC: head circumference)

larger HC than when measured in TT plane, studies have found that it is not clinically relevant.[2] As TT plane is more commonly used in most parts of the world, it is important to identify the landmarks of this plane on ultrasound.

Transthalamic plane is a cross-sectional view of fetal head obtained at the level of thalami which are located symmetrically on either side of midline **(Fig. 2)**. The image should be as close as possible to horizontal with an angle of insonation close to 90°. There is a centrally positioned, continuous midline echo (falx cerebri) which is broken anteriorly at one third of its length by a box-shaped structure, i.e., cavum septum pellucidum (CSP). In a true axial image, the calvarium and intracranial structures appear symmetric on either side of midline. To avoid errors in measurement, both frontal and occipital bones should be clearly visible. Also, orbits and posterior fossa should not be visible in the image. The image should be appropriately magnified such that fetal head fills up 50% of monitor screen.

Step 2: Placement of Calipers

Two methods have been described to measure BPD—outer-to-inner caliper placement and outer-to-outer caliper placement. In outer-to-inner caliper placement, caliper which is closer to the ultrasound transducer, i.e., at the top of image, is placed at the outer edge of proximal parietal bone of skull, while the distal caliper is placed at the inner edge of distal parietal bone at the widest part of skull. In outer-to-outer caliper placement, both proximal and distal calipers are placed at the outer edges of proximal and distal parietal bones at the widest part of skull. Studies have shown that using modern ultrasound equipment, both the above methods are equally reproducible. However, the correct chart should be used depending upon method used for caliper placement while assigning gestational age based on BPD.

For measuring HC, ellipse calipers are commonly used such that the line of ellipse runs along the outer edge of skull.

Head circumference can also be calculated with the help of BPD and occipitofrontal diameter (OFD) using the formula HC = 1.62 × (BPD + OFD).[3] OFD is commonly measured as distance between caliper placed at outer edge of anterior frontal wall and caliper placed at outer edge of distal occipital wall at the longest part of skull. A study by Napolitano et al. found that measurement of HC using ellipse facility is marginally more reproducible than using BPD and OFD for the same.[2] This is probably because OFD is the least reproducible head measurement on ultrasound.

ABDOMINAL MEASUREMENTS

Three abdominal measurements have been described for assessment of fetal growth. These include AC, anteroposterior abdominal diameter (APAD), and transverse abdominal diameter (TAD). All three are taken in the same ultrasound view. AC using ellipse is the most used measurement out of the three. It

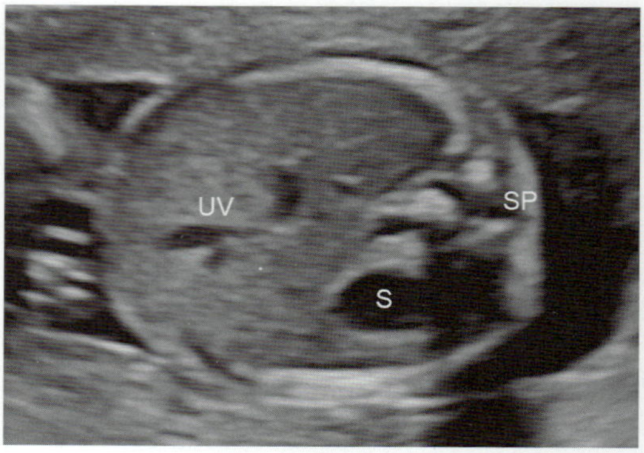

Fig. 3: Axial image of fetal abdomen used for measuring AC. Stomach (S) and short segment of UV can be seen with a single rib visible on each side. (AC: abdominal circumference; SP: spine; UV: umbilical vein)

is measured in a transverse section of fetal abdomen as close as possible to circular. Landmarks to be noted are spine with a single, symmetrical rib on each side. Outer skin surface should preferably be visible all around. In the correct plane, stomach bubble and short segment of umbilical vein are visible **(Fig. 3)**. If the entire intra-abdominal umbilical vein is seen, it implies that the plane is too angled and will lead to measurement error.[4] Also, if a part of kidney is visible, it signifies that the image is too low in the abdomen for correct measurement. The operator should avoid applying too much pressure with the ultrasound transducer so as to not distort the circular shape of fetal abdomen. The image should be appropriately magnified so that fetal abdomen fills at least 30% of monitor screen. Placement of calipers should be such that the ellipse runs along the outer border of abdomen (outer surface of skin).

FEMUR LENGTH MEASUREMENT

Measurement of FL involves measurement of ossified femoral diaphysis **(Fig. 4)**. Femur

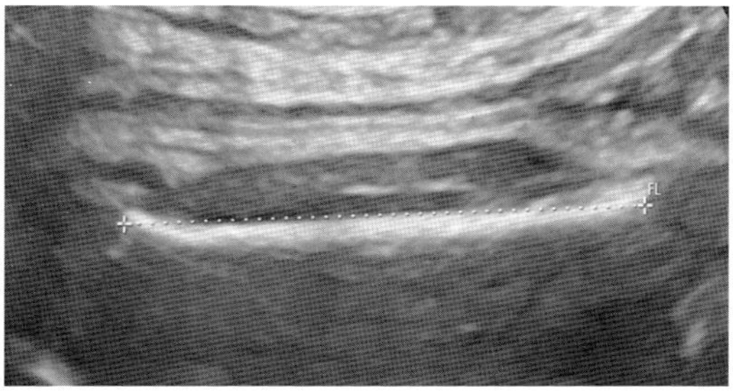

Fig. 4: Ossified femoral diaphysis for measurement of femur length (FL).

which is closest to the ultrasound probe is chosen for measurement. For accurate measurement, femur should be as close as possible to horizontal plane with an angle of insonation close to 90°. Image should be appropriately magnified so that cross-section of femur fills at least 50% of monitor screen. Calipers should be placed on the outer border of edges of femoral diaphysis. Care should be taken not to include the greater trochanter and femoral epiphyses while placing calipers to avoid overestimation of FL.

ESTIMATED FETAL WEIGHT

Estimated fetal weight is often used to monitor fetal growth trends prenatally and to counsel parents regarding anticipated birth weight in case delivery is planned. It is important to note that EFW is measurement of fetal size at a particular point of time and does not describe fetal growth which is dynamic. For correct interpretation of fetal growth, longitudinal growth charts are needed to evaluate fetal growth velocity over multiple visits.

Several formulas have been developed for assessing EFW that incorporate measurements of fetal head, abdomen, and FL. The most widely used formula is the one published by Hadlock et al. in 1985.[5] An important pitfall with the use of EFW is that errors in measurement of individual parameters may get amplified. Therefore, every effort should be made to obtain the best possible measurement. This is especially important for AC which can be difficult to measure accurately because of technical factors.

Once EFW is calculated, it is generally plotted against reference EFW for that gestation to identify fetuses who are at risk of adverse pregnancy outcomes (SGA or LGA). Growth charts which are commonly used include the one described by Hadlock et al. in 1991, the World Health Organization (WHO) fetal growth charts, and INTERGROWTH-21st growth charts.[6,7]

BIOMETRY REPORTING

Ultrasound measurements can be reported as raw data (in mm or cm), in terms of weeks of pregnancy, in terms of centiles, or in the form of Z scores. The last two methods help the obstetrician and patient to understand deviation from mean of a standard reference population at any given gestational age. Centiles are easy to understand and cutoff point below 10th centile for gestation for AC and/or EFW have been incorporated into definitions of fetal growth restriction.[8] Also, serial measurements of individual fetal parameters and EFW give more information than single size measurement as they help to understand fetal growth velocity rather than fetal size. Hence, wherever possible, fetal biometry should be expressed in centiles and serial measurements should be plotted on growth chart for better understanding of fetal growth.

DOPPLER

Doppler ultrasound, when performed correctly, is a very important tool in the hands of the operator to assess fetal well-being and identifying fetuses who may be at risk of adverse pregnancy outcomes. During Doppler imaging, thermal index (TI) and mechanical index (MI) should be displayed on monitor screen (TI and MI should be ≤1.0) and scanning time with Doppler should be kept as short as possible. ALARA (as low as reasonably achievable) principle should be followed during examination. To study maternal and fetal circulation, three Doppler modalities are commonly used—color Doppler, power Doppler, and spectral Doppler. Knowledge about gain settings and pulse repetition frequency (PRF) helps to improve the information obtained from Doppler technology. PRF refers to the frequency at which ultrasound signals are emitted. With low PRF, signals from slow-moving targets (like low-velocity blood vessels) can be studied. High PRF is beneficial in studying high-velocity blood flow.

Color Doppler

While using color Doppler, size of the color box should be kept as small as possible to include the study area only. PRF should be adjusted according to the blood flow velocity in vessel being studied. For studying low-velocity vessels, PRF may need to be reduced, while high-velocity vessels may require PRF to be increased to avoid aliasing. Conventionally, flow toward the transducer is shown as red, while flow away from transducer is shown as blue.

Power Doppler

Power Doppler is more sensitive than color Doppler when studying low-velocity blood flow. It is less dependent on angle of insonation than color Doppler.

Spectral Pulsed Wave Doppler

Spectral Doppler is commonly used to study maternal and fetal circulation. Recording of waveform is preferred at the time of fetal quiescence (in the absence of fetal breathing and body movements). Temporary maternal breath holding may also be beneficial in some cases. For optimal measurements, angle of insonation should be as close to zero as possible, i.e., with insonation aligned with the direction of blood flow. This is critically important when measuring MCA peak systolic velocity (MCA-PSV) to identify cases with fetal anemia. Doppler gate (sample volume) needs to be adjusted according to the width of vessel being studied. For example, a narrow Doppler gate is used while studying DV at the time of 11–13 weeks ultrasound, while a relatively wide Doppler gate is used to study umbilical artery in third trimester. By convention, flow toward the ultrasound transducer is displayed as waveforms above the baseline, while flow away from transducer is displayed as waveforms below the baseline. An average of indices of three consecutive waveforms obtained during Doppler recording is used for reporting.

Doppler indices that are commonly used in obstetric practice are:

- *Pulsatility index:* (Peak systolic velocity – minimum diastolic velocity)/mean velocity
- *Resistance index (RI):* (Peak systolic velocity – minimum diastolic velocity)/peak systolic velocity
- Peak systolic velocity
- *Cerebroplacental ratio (CPR):* MCA PI/UA PI

It was in 2016 that Delphi consensus definition of FGR was published by Gordijn et al.[8] Since then, ultrasound measurements focusing on Doppler waveform analysis of fetal circulation (UA, MCA, and DV) and maternal circulation (uterine artery) have been widely incorporated into obstetric practice.

UMBILICAL ARTERY

In a normal pregnancy, there is an increase in end-diastolic flow in UA with advancing gestation due to increase in tertiary stem villi that occurs with maturation of placenta **(Fig. 5A)**. UA Doppler waveform can be obtained at different sites in the umbilical cord. These include placental end of cord, fetal end of cord, or free loop. Resistance in UA is highest at fetal end of cord insertion and lowest at placental end. Because of this, absent end-diastolic flow/reversed end-diastolic flow (REDF) is most likely to be seen first at fetal end of umbilical cord. For the sake of consistency, the International Society of Ultrasound in Obstetrics and Gynecology (ISUOG) recommends measuring UA waveforms from a free loop of cord.[9] Abnormal Doppler waveform in UA reflects downstream resistance in placental circulation which can occur in cases of placental pathology. The progression of abnormal UA waveforms can be seen on ultrasound in the form of decreased end-diastolic flow (increased PI) which can progress to absent end-diastolic flow **(Fig. 5B)** or REDF **(Fig. 5C)**. REDF has been shown to be associated with adverse perinatal outcome independent of prematurity.[10]

MIDDLE CEREBRAL ARTERY

For assessment of middle cerebral artery, a low axial section of brain is obtained at the level of wings of sphenoid bone. On adding color Doppler, circle of Willis and proximal MCA are identified. Pulsed wave Doppler gate is then placed on the proximal third of MCA close to its origin. Angle of insonation should be kept as close to 0° as possible (ultrasound beam should be aligned with the

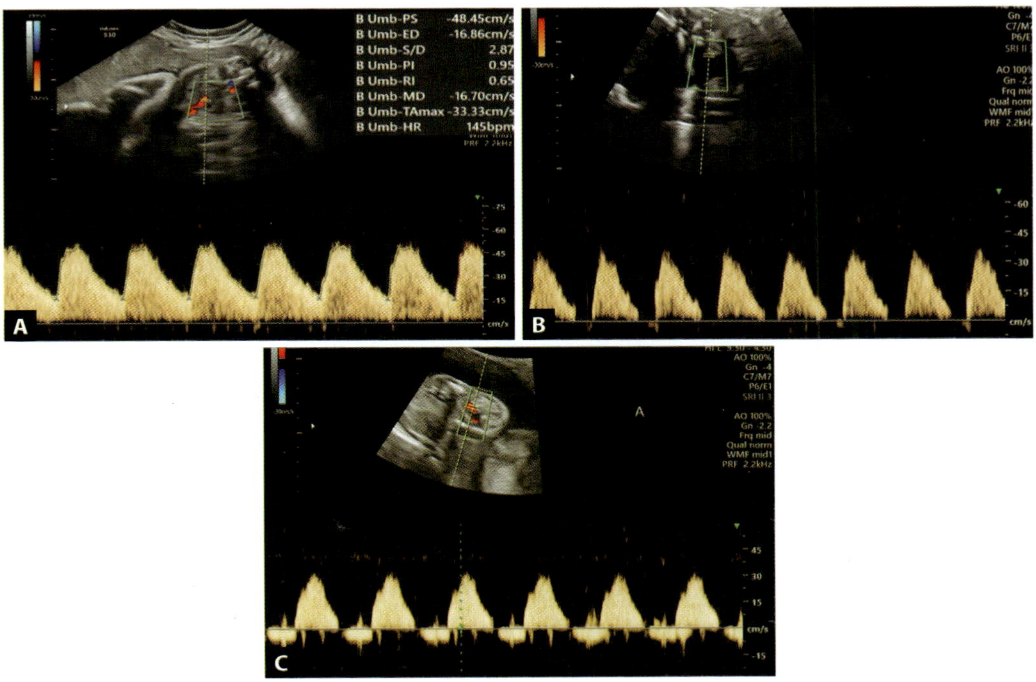

Figs. 5A to C: Umbilical artery (UA) Doppler waveforms: (A) Normal UA Doppler; (B) Absent end-diastolic flow (AEDF) in UA; (C) Reversed end-diastolic flow (REDF) in UA.

direction of blood flow in MCA). Unnecessary pressure on fetal head can lead to erroneous decrease in end-diastolic velocity (EDV), increase in PSV, and PI and hence should be avoided. For MCA-PSV measurement, distal MCA can be used if 0° angle of insonation is easier to obtain for distal MCA compared to proximal MCA.

Middle cerebral artery normally shows high impedance flow with continuous forward flow throughout the cardiac cycle **(Fig. 6A)**. In case of fetal hypoxemia, MCA responds to changes in oxygen tension with increase in diastolic blood flow which is reflected in decrease in PI of MCA **(Fig. 6B)**. MCA-PSV >1.5 multiple of the median is a marker for fetal anemia.

CEREBROPLACENTAL RATIO

Cerebroplacental ratio is calculated by dividing MCA PI by UA PI. CPR improves the sensitivity of UA and MCA Doppler. In cases with mild increase in placental resistance and mild decrease in fetal brain vascular resistance, UA PI and MCA PI may be within normal range, but CPR will be decreased. CPR is often already abnormal when UA and MCA depict mild changes in Doppler waveforms. While interpreting CPR, gestational age-based reference charts should be used rather than a single cutoff. In the Delphi consensus definition of FGR, CPR <5th centile is one of the criteria used for diagnosing late-onset FGR.[8]

DUCTUS VENOSUS

Ductus venosus is a narrow vessel which connects intra-abdominal portion of umbilical vein to inferior vena cava just below the diaphragm. It is a shunt in fetal life which preferentially directs oxygen-rich blood in umbilical vein to fetal heart, bypassing the liver. It can be visualized in two planes—either in sagittal longitudinal plane of fetal trunk or in an oblique transverse plane through fetal abdomen. On applying color Doppler, high-velocity blood flow in this narrow vessel can be appreciated in the form of aliasing. Sample gate needs to be adjusted according to period of gestation. A narrow sample gate often helps to get a clear recording of flow in DV. Waveform in DV is normally triphasic **(Fig. 7A)**. Waveform deflection during atrial contraction ("a" wave) and DV PI are used in evaluation of fetuses with FGR and help to guide delivery decisions. With evolving placental dysfunction, "a" wave may go down to the baseline (absent "a" wave) or may even

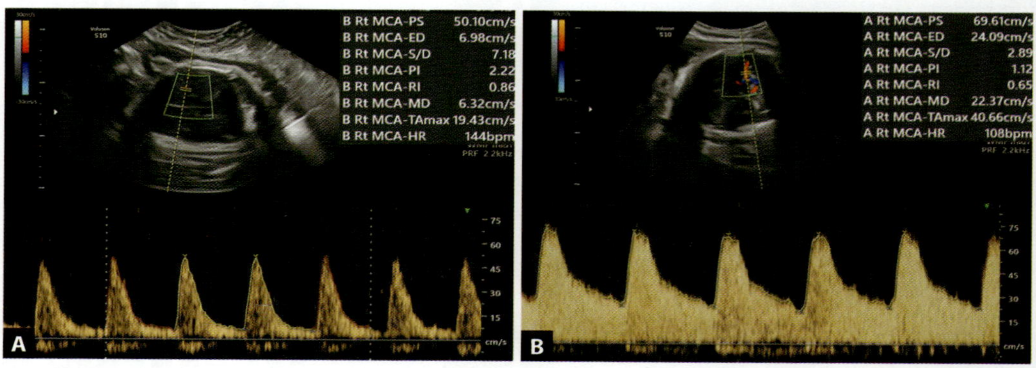

Figs. 6A and B: Middle cerebral artery (MCA) Doppler waveforms: (A) Normal high impedance flow in MCA and (B) increased diastolic flow in MCA due to low impedance in cerebral circulation (brain-sparing effect).

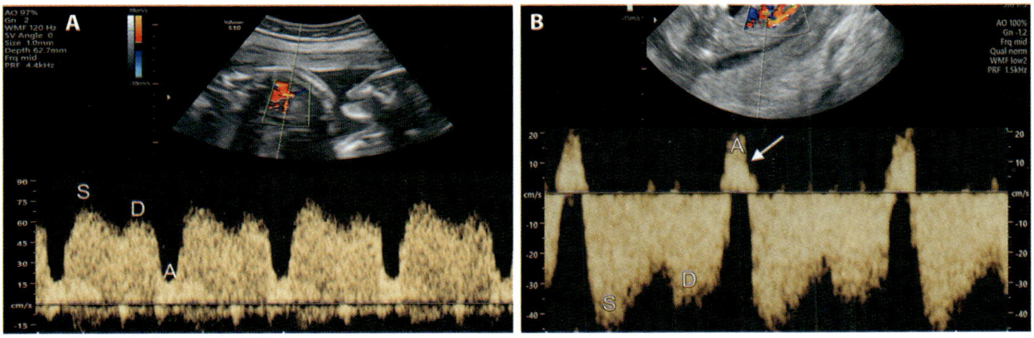

Figs. 7A and B: Ductus venosus (DV) Doppler waveforms: (A) Triphasic DV Doppler waveform (S corresponds to ventricular systole, D corresponds to early diastole, and A corresponds to late diastole or atrial kick). (B) Reversal of "a" wave (arrow) in DV.

go below the baseline or reverse (reversal of "a" wave) **(Fig. 7B)**. Reversal of "a" wave in DV is thought to be a sign of cardiac dysfunction or fetal acidemia. It is important not to confuse hepatic vein with DV. Hepatic veins also have a S, D, and a wave, but velocities are lower and it is normal to have "a" wave reversal in hepatic vein.

UTERINE ARTERY

In 1983, Campbell et al. used pulsed Doppler to study blood flow pattern in arcuate vessels in second and third trimesters of pregnancy. They proposed that this technique can give early warning for impaired uteroplacental perfusion. In the last 10–15 years, there has been a resurgence in interest in uterine artery Doppler study in late pregnancy. Unlike Campbell et al. who studied arcuate vessels, studies done over the last decade have focused on Doppler ultrasound study of main branch of uterine artery.

Techniques to assess uterine artery Doppler are:

- First-trimester uterine artery Doppler assessment is generally done by imaging sagittal section of uterus. Cervical canal and internal os are identified. Ultrasound transducer is then gently tilted from side to side and uterine artery is identified at the level of internal os by color flow mapping. By keeping the sample gate at 2 mm, uterine artery waveform is studied with pulsed Doppler. When imaged correctly, PSV in uterine artery should be above 60 cm/s.
- In the second and third trimester, ultrasound probe is placed in iliac fossa and angled medially. With the help of color Doppler, uterine artery is identified as it crosses over the hypogastric artery and vein. Sample volume of pulsed Doppler is placed 1 cm above the crossover point such that angle with the direction of blood flow is <30°.

Trophoblastic invasion of spiral arteries during pregnancy transforms them into low-resistance vessels to ensure continuous blood supply to intervillous space **(Fig. 8A)**. Defective trophoblastic infusion is thought to increase the risk for preeclampsia and FGR. Uterine artery may show increased PI and early-diastolic notch in such cases **(Fig. 8B)**. In the Delphi consensus definition of early-onset FGR, uterine artery PI >95th centile is one of the criteria used for diagnosing early-onset FGR.

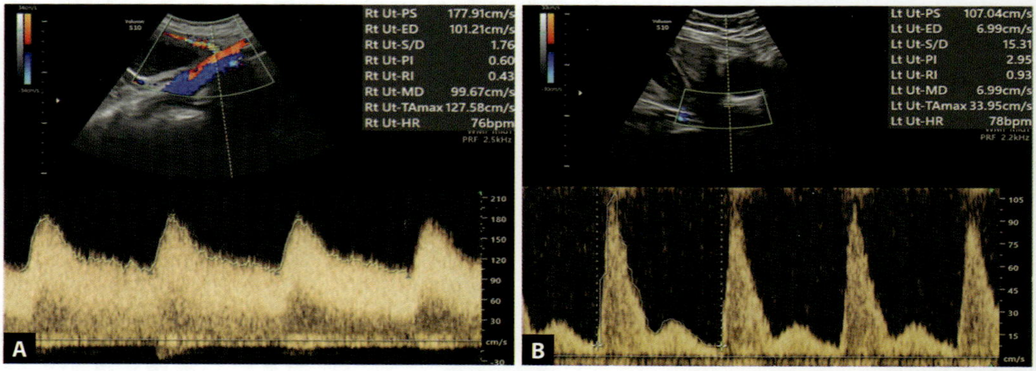

Figs. 8A and B: Uterine artery Doppler waveforms: (A) Normal low-resistance uterine artery Doppler waveform; (B) Abnormal uterine artery Doppler with early-diastolic notch and increased pulsatility index (PI).

REFERENCES

1. Hadlock FP, Shah YP, Kanon DJ, Lindsey JV. Fetal crown-rump length: reevaluation of relation to menstrual age (5-18 weeks) with high resolution real-time US. Radiology. 1992;182:501-5.
2. Napolitano R, Donadono V, Ohuma EO, Knight CL, Wanyonyi SZ, Kemp B, et al. Scientific basis for standardization of fetal head measurements by ultrasound: a reproducibility study. Ultrasound Obstet Gynecol. 2016;48(1):80-5.
3. Salomon LJ, Alfirevic Z, Berghella V, Bilardo C, Hernandez-Andrade E, Johnsen SL, et al. Practice guidelines for performance of the routine mid-trimester fetal ultrasound scan. Ultrasound Obstet Gynecol. 2010;37: 116-26.
4. The International Fetal and Newborn Growth Consortium. (2009). The International Fetal and Newborn Growth Standards for the 21st Century (INTERGROWTH-21st) Study Protocol. [online] Available from https://www.medscinet.net/Intergrowth/patientinfodocs/Intergrowth%20Protocol%20Sept%202009.pdf [Last accessed March, 2024].
5. Hadlock FP, Harrist RB, Sharman RS, Deter RL, Park SK. Estimation of fetal weight with the use of head, body, and femur measurements: a prospective study. Am J Obstet Gynecol. 1985;151:333-7.
6. Papageorghiou AT, Ohuma EO, Altman DG, Todros T, Ismail LC, Lambert A, et al. International standards for fetal growth based on serial ultrasound measurements: The Fetal Growth Longitudinal Study of the INTERGROWTH-21st Project. Lancet. 2014;384:869-79.
7. Kiserud T, Piaggio G, Carroli G, Widmer M, Carvalho J, Neerup Jensen L, et al. The World Health Organization Fetal Growth Charts: A Multinational Longitudinal Study of Ultrasound Biometric Measurements and Estimated Fetal Weight. PLoS Med. 2017;14(1):e1002220.
8. Gordijn SJ, Beune IM, Thilaganathan B, Papageorghiou A, Baschat AA, Baker PN, et al. Consensus definition of fetal growth restriction: a Delphi procedure. Ultrasound Obstet Gynecol. 2016;48:333-9.
9. Bhide A, Acharya G, Baschat A, Bilardo CM, Brezinka C, Cafici D, et al. ISUOG Practice Guidelines (updated): use of Doppler velocimetry in obstetrics. Ultrasound Obstet Gynecol. 2021;58:331-9.
10. Figueras F, Gratacós E. Update on the diagnosis and classification of fetal growth restriction and proposal of a stage-based management protocol. Fetal Diagn Ther. 2014;36(2):86-98.

CHAPTER

6

Genetic Sonogram: How to Interpret Soft Markers

Vandana Chaddha, Nikhil Kapoor, Shilpa Thakur

KEY POINTS

1. Soft markers are sonographic findings that typically reflect normal variation in fetal anatomy but are associated with a small-to-moderate increased risk of aneuploidy.
2. Absence of markers has been associated with a 50–80% reduction in the maternal age-related risk, thus providing the parents with information that could be used to make informed choices on whether to pursue diagnostic–genetic testing.
3. Presence of a single marker like echogenic foci, renal pelviectasis, choroid plexus cyst (CPC), and aberrant right subclavian artery, in the background of normal cell-free deoxyribonucleic acid (DNA) screen, is not considered clinically significant and may not warrant invasive testing.
4. Presence of markers such as thickened nuchal fold, ventriculomegaly, short long bones need further testing as these are associated with high likelihood ratio of aneuploidy hence warrant invasive test for confirmation.
5. Aneuploidy is rare in a fetus with an isolated marker after a detailed anatomic survey, and chromosomal analysis is not typically performed when no other malformations or indications for genetic amniocentesis are present **(Table 1)**.
6. The incidence of growth restriction also varies with the type of aneuploidy. Among fetuses with trisomy 21, 13, and 18, growth restriction has been reported in 30%, 50%, and 90% of cases, respectively.
7. A low-risk result on cell-free DNA screening may be falsely reassuring in the setting of a structural anomaly.

TABLE 1: Summary of soft markers in the first and second trimesters.

A	First-trimester soft markers	• Enlarged NT • Early fetal lymphangiectasia • First-trimester absent nasal bone • Megacystis • First-trimester growth restriction
B	Second-trimester soft markers	• Echogenic intracardiac focus • CPCs • SUA • Urinary tract dilation • Slightly shortened long bones (humerus, femur) • Hyperechoic bowel • Thickened nuchal fold • Absent or hypoplastic nasal bone • Aberrant right subclavian artery

(CPC: choroid plexus cyst; NT: nuchal translucency; SUA: single umbilical artery)

INTRODUCTION

Aneuploidy is the most common genetic abnormality detected by prenatal diagnosis.

The antepartum detection of fetal aneuploidy is one of the major goals of prenatal screening programs **(Box 1)**.

SCREENING MODALITIES FOR GENETIC DISEASE/ ANEUPLOIDIES

Screening modalities for genetic disease/ aneuploidies are as follows:

- Assessing parental risk factors for genetic disease which includes age as well as history of previous affected babies.
- Maternal cell-free deoxyribonucleic acid
- Biomarker screening
- Sonographic findings mainly soft markers and some specific congenital anomalies associated with aneuploides.

Definition of soft markers: Soft markers are sonographic findings that typically reflect normal variation in fetal anatomy but are associated with a small-to-moderate increased risk of aneuploidy. They may be transient, resolving with advancing gestational age or after birth, often with no clinical sequelae.[1]

BOX 1: Common aneuploidies according to European surveillance of congenital anomalies database.

- Trisomy 21
- Trisomy 18
- Trisomy 13
- XXX
- XXY
- XYY
- XO

Definitive genetic diagnosis can be done by confirmatory invasive tests:

- Amniocentesis
- Chorionic villus sampling
- Fetal blood
- Fetal tissue sampling

First Trimester

Nuchal translucency (NT) at 11 + 0 to 13 + 6 weeks **(Figs. 1A and B)**.

Criteria

Nuchal translucency: It is the clear space at the posterior aspect of fetal neck, between the spine and the skin edge.

Sonographic features: Fetal midsagittal plane; crown–rump length (CRL) is 45–84 mm (approximately 11–14 weeks of gestation).

Enlarged NT definition: Measuring ≥3.5 mm or ≥95th or 99th percentile for gestational age by CRL.

Providers performing NT measurement: They should be appropriately qualified and the program should be audited.

Relevance

Enlarged NT may be associated with the following:

- Atypical chromosomal abnormalities (e.g., deletion, duplication, unbalanced

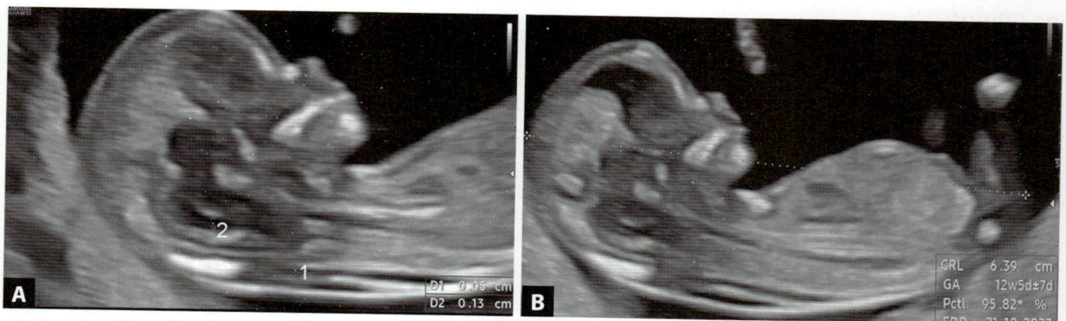

Figs. 1A and B: Normal nuchal translucency (NT) and nasal bone seen at 12 weeks of gestational age (GA). (CRL: crown–rump length)

structural rearrangement, mosaicism, and rare autosomal trisomy)

- Submicroscopic aberrations
- Single-gene disorders including RASopathies
- Structural malformations

As NT becomes progressively larger, the risk of fetal aneuploidy and other adverse outcomes (e.g., structural abnormalities, particularly congenital heart disease) increases.

Disappearance of an enlarged NT prior to 14 weeks gestation occurs in approximately 20% fetuses and is associated with an improved prognosis.[2]

Early Fetal Lymphangiectasia (Enlarged Nuchal Region/Edema at 9–10 Weeks)

Criteria

Definition: NT >95th percentile for CRL 28–44 mm or >2.2 mm, but there is limited data to establish these criteria.

Relevance

In contrast to enlarged NT at 11 + 0 to 13 + 6 weeks, the significance of lymphangiectasia (fetal edema) or thickened nuchal region at 9–10 weeks of gestation (CRL <45 mm) is not clearly established. In this case, patients can be offered cell-free DNA screening. A repeat scan should be performed at 11–14 weeks; if NT is enlarged, then diagnostic testing should be offered.[3]

Cystic Hygroma

Criteria

Cystic hygroma is singular or multiloculated fluid collection, which typically occurs along the posterior fetal neck and back.

Relevance

Cause: It occurs due to abnormal lymphatic development with delayed communication between the lymphatic and vascular systems. However, communication may subsequently occur, resulting in reversal of this finding.

Cystic hygroma is associated with a substantially increased risk of:

- Autosomal trisomy (50–60%)
- Copy number variants
- RASopathies (e.g., Noonan syndrome)
- Monosomy X (Turner syndrome; 45, X)
- In euploid fetuses, 30–50% have structural anomalies (cardiac malformations common).[4]

First-trimester Absent Nasal Bone

Criteria

When the fetal profile is viewed in the midsagittal plane, the nasal bone appears as an echogenic line within the bridge of the nose, under the skin edge. The nasal bone is considered present if this line is more echogenic than the overlying skin and absent if it is not visualized or less echogenic than the overlying skin **(Figs. 2A and B)**.

Relevance

The frequency of an absent nasal bone in euploid, trisomy 13, trisomy 18, and trisomy 21 fetuses was 2.5%, 45%, 53%, and 60%, respectively. In a euploid fetus, a nonvisualized nasal bone may reflect delayed maturation, rather than the true absence of the nasal bone, and is reported in 4.7% of euploid fetuses with a CRL of 45–54 mm, progressively decreasing to 1% in those with a CRL of 74–84 mm.[5]

Megacystis (An Enlarged Fetal Bladder)

Criteria

Longitudinal bladder length ≥7 mm at 10–14 weeks of gestation.

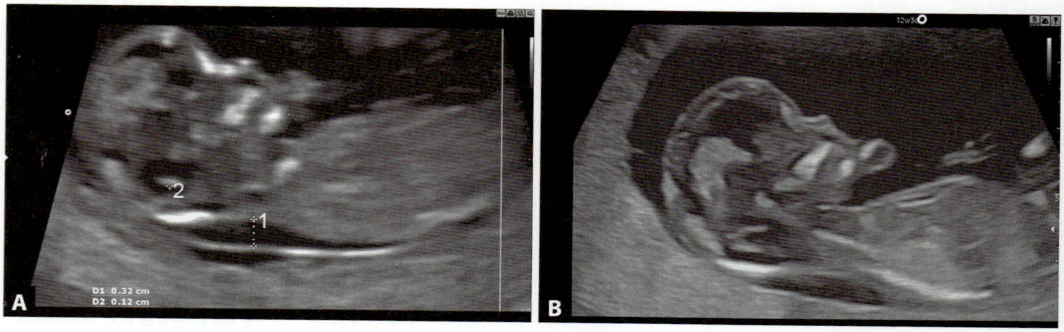

Figs. 2A and B: Abnormal nuchal translucency/nasal bone (NT/NB) scan for a fetus at comparable gestation.

Relevance

Incidence: 1 in 1,500 pregnancies.

Associations:

- Chromosomal abnormalities
- Genetic syndromes
- Anomalies of the urinary tract
- Resolve spontaneously with good outcome

In a retrospective cohort study of 98 patients; aneuploidy rate with megacystis are as follows:

- Trisomy 18: 50%
- Trisomy 13: 25%
- Trisomy 21: 25%

If isolated megacystis and NT measurement <95th percentile, no cases of aneuploidy were identified, and majority had resolution of the megacystis.

Livebirths with resolution of the megacystis:

- 80% had normal outcome
- 6% had vertebral defects, anal atresia, cardiac defects, tracheoesophageal fistula, renal anomalies, and limb abnormalities (VACTERL) or imperforate anus/fistula
- 14% had other urologic diagnoses
- No cases of lower urinary tract obstruction among fetuses with a bladder length <12 mm.[6]

First-trimester Growth Restriction

Criteria

If the dating scan has been satisfactorily performed, then the criteria for growth delay are established when the CRL on a subsequent first-trimester ultrasound examination performed at least 7–14 days later indicates a gestational age that is >5–7 days younger than expected by the initial ultrasound examination.

Relevance

The severity of growth restriction correlates with the severity of the chromosomal abnormality. The association between short CRL and aneuploidy was strong for trisomy 18 and 13 and triploidy but not observed for trisomy 21.[7]

First-trimester Doppler markers for aneuploidy screening ***(Figs. 3 and 4)***

- *Abnormal flow in the ductus venosus:* In one review, the frequency of reversed a wave in the ductus venosus by karyotype was 3% for euploid fetuses, 55% for trisomy 13, 58% for trisomy 18, and 66% for trisomy 21.
- *Tricuspid regurgitation:* It may be seen in both aneuploid and euploid fetuses. In one study, the frequency of tricuspid regurgitation at 11–13 weeks by karyotype was 0.9% for euploid fetuses, 55.7% for trisomy 21, 33.3% for trisomy 18, 30% for trisomy 13, and 37.5% for monosomy X. As an isolated finding, it is a poor screening tool for aneuploidy and congenital heart defects.[5]

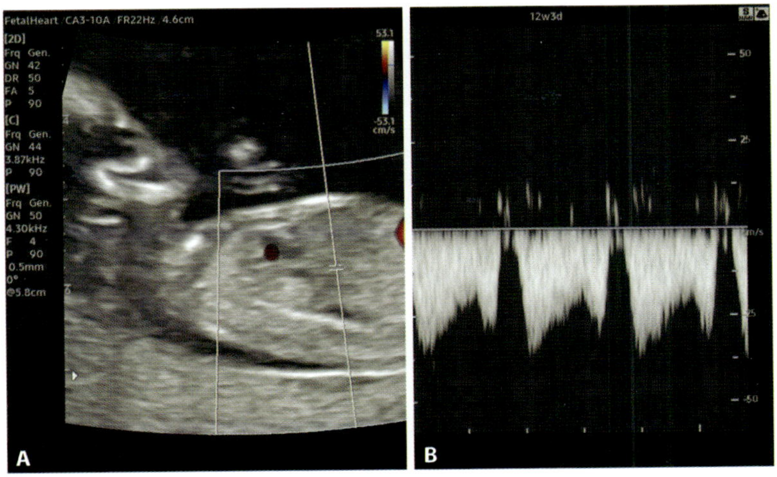

Figs. 3A and B: Absent a wave in ductus venosus in a diagnosed case of aneuploidy.

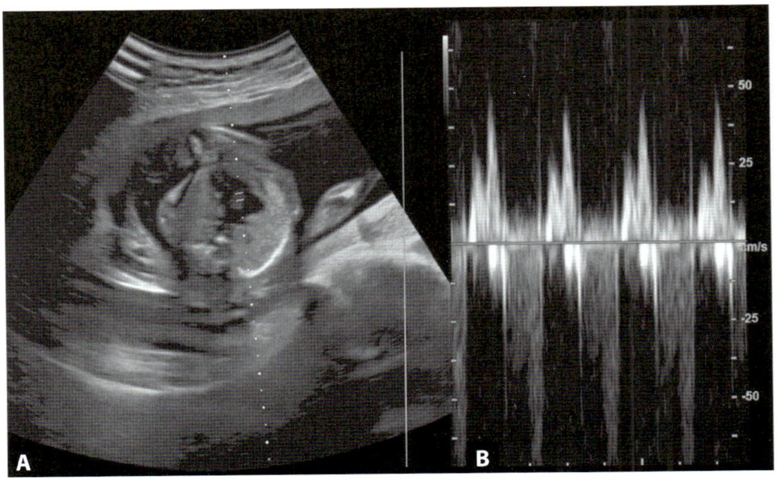

Figs. 4A and B: Tricuspid regurgitation in prenatally diagnosed Down syndrome.

Second-trimester Soft Markers

Echogenic Intracardiac Focus (Fig. 5)

Criteria: An echogenic intracardiac focus (EIF) is a punctate echogenic area that is typically seen in the left cardiac ventricle but may be seen in either or both ventricles. To be considered an EIF, it must be as bright as bone and seen in two imaging planes.

Relevance: Echogenic intracardiac focuses are not associated with myocardial dysfunction or structural cardiac anomalies. An isolated EIF in the setting of an otherwise normal detailed structural survey is considered a normal variant in the setting of a low-risk cell-free DNA screen.

Choroid Plexus Cysts

Criteria

Choroid plexus cysts are typically small (<10 mm in diameter) sonolucent structures

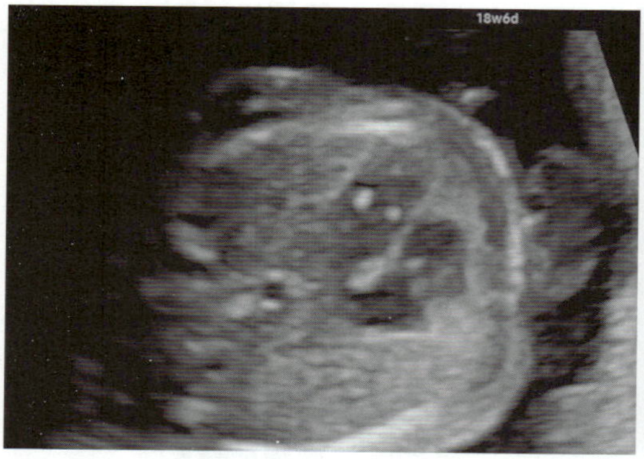

Fig. 5: Echogenic foci in a case of Down syndrome with aberrant right subclavian artery.

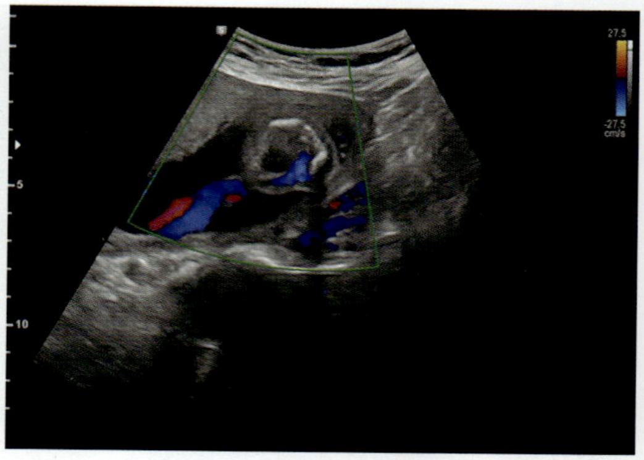

Fig. 6: Single umbilical artery.

with well-delineated borders within the choroid plexus of the cerebral lateral ventricles. They may be unilateral single simple cysts to septate, bilateral, or multiple cysts.

Relevance

Isolated CPCs in the setting of an otherwise normal detailed obstetrical ultrasound and low-risk aneuploidy screening are considered a normal variant. They are not associated with adverse long-term developmental outcomes. Those that persist beyond the second trimester are typically asymptomatic and benign.

Single Umbilical Artery (Fig. 6)

Criteria

Prenatal diagnosis of single umbilical artery (SUA) is based on ultrasound examination showing two instead of three vessels in the umbilical cord (cross section or longitudinally). Color flow Doppler in the region of the bifurcation of the fetal aorta shows intra-abdominal umbilical vessels on only one side of the fetal bladder which is pathognomonic of SUA.

Relevance

Aneuploidy is rare in a fetus with an isolated SUA after a detailed anatomic survey, and chromosomal analysis is not typically performed when no other malformations or indications for genetic amniocentesis are present.

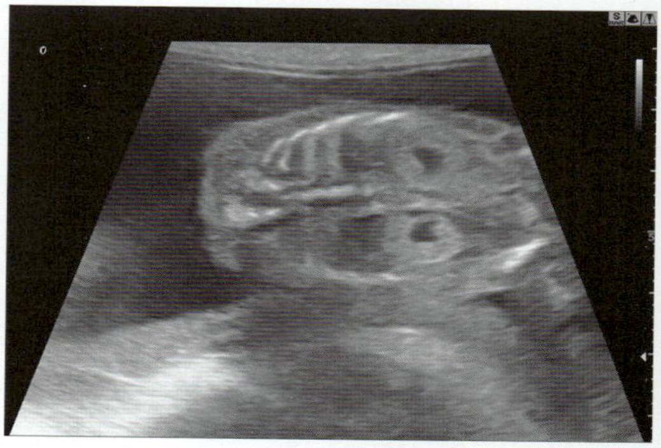

Fig. 7: Urinary tract dilatation in a second-trimester fetus with Down syndrome.

Urinary Tract Dilatation (Fig. 7)

Criteria

Mild (grade 1) antenatal (A) urinary tract dilation (UTD-A1; previously known as mild pyelectasis), is usually defined as a renal pelvic diameter of 4 to <7 mm pelvic dilation at 16–27 weeks of gestation.

Relevance

Urinary tract dilation A1 is seen in 1–2% of fetuses overall, but 11–17% of fetuses with trisomy 21. However, the presence of both a detailed anatomic survey and a low-risk cell-free DNA screen for fetal aneuploidy is reassuring.

For fetuses with more severe UTD (antenatally categorized as UTD-A2 or 3), follow-up imaging and care should be individualized based on sonographic features and clinical circumstance.

Slightly Short Long Bones

Criteria

Various criteria have been published for determining whether a femur or humerus is short with respect to aneuploidy screening. The criteria are usually based on observed-to-expected ratios or multiple of the median with respect to biparietal diameter (BPD) <0.9 to be abnormal. It can also be defined as the femoral length below the 5th centile for gestational age (some define it as below the 2.5th centile).

The femur must be measured meticulously with an angle of insonation perpendicular to the bone and the calipers at the end of the diaphysis.

Significance

A slightly short femur is detected in approximately 28% of fetuses with trisomy 21 and 6% are euploid fetuses. A shortened humerus is a slightly better predictor of trisomy 21 than a shortened femur (positive likelihood ratios of 4.8 and 3.7, respectively). These two markers often occur in conjunction with each other.

In contrast, a very short femur (<5th percentile) or abnormal appearing long bones may be a sign of a skeletal dysplasia, early onset fetal growth restriction (FGR), and presence of pathogenic copy number variants.[8]

Echogenic Bowel (Hyperechoic Bowel) (Fig. 8)

Criteria

Fetal hyperechoic bowel refers to increased echogenicity (brightness) of the fetal bowel noted on second-trimester sonographic examination. To be considered hyperechoic, the bowel must be as bright as bone using a transabdominal transducer with a frequency of ≤5 MHz, with harmonics turned off and lower gain.

Significance

Hyperechoic bowel is seen in 13–21% of fetuses with trisomy 21 and 1–2% of euploid fetuses. In fetuses with hyperechoic bowel, trisomy 21 is the most common aneuploidy identified. Isolated hyperechoic bowel has been reported with sex chromosome aneuploidies, which are potentially detectable with cell-free DNA screening.

Hyperechoic bowel is transient, regressing or disappearing in up to 72% of fetuses but it also can be associated with the following complications: Cystic fibrosis, congenital infection, intra-amniotic bleeding, fetal growth restriction, and gastrointestinal pathology.

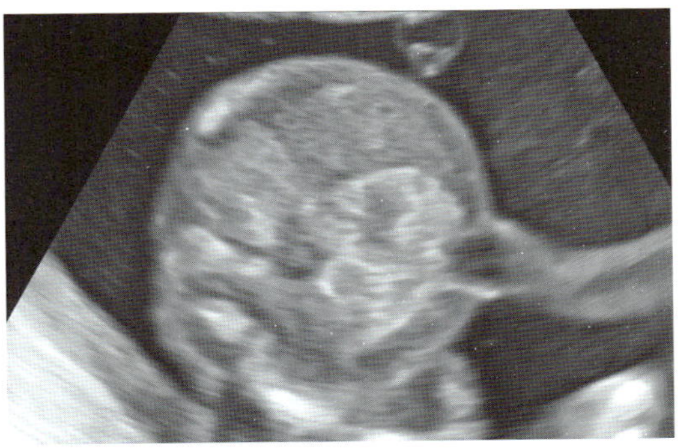

Fig. 8: Echogenic bowel in a second-trimester fetus.

Thick Nuchal Fold (Fig. 9)

Criteria

The nuchal fold refers to the skin in the back of the fetal neck evaluated in the second trimester. The skin thickness is measured in an axial plane of the fetal head where the cavum septi pellucidum, thalami, cerebral peduncles, and cerebellar hemispheres are demonstrated. The measurement is made from the outer edge occipital bone to the skin edge. A nuchal fold is considered thick if the measurement is ≥6 mm.

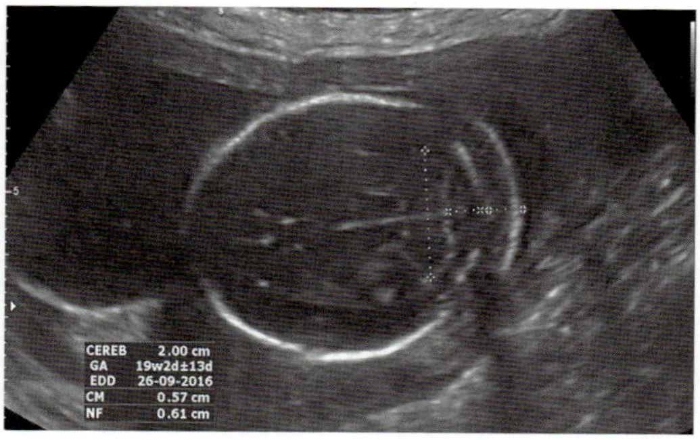

Fig. 9: Thick nuchal fold in case of Down syndrome.

Significance

Increased thickness of the nuchal fold is one of the most sensitive markers for trisomy 21 in the second trimester, detected in at least 20–50% fetuses with trisomy 21 and 0.5–2% euploid fetuses. As an isolated finding, it carries a likelihood ratio for trisomy 21 of between 3 and 11.

A thick nuchal fold has also been observed with sex chromosome abnormalities.[8]

Second-trimester Absent Nasal Bone (Figs. 10A to C)

Criteria

Methods proposed: Nasal bone length of ≤2.5 mm or a gestational age threshold of <2.5th or 5th percentile or <0.75 multiples of the median for gestational age.

Significance

In the second trimester, the nasal bone is absent in approximately 30–40% fetuses with

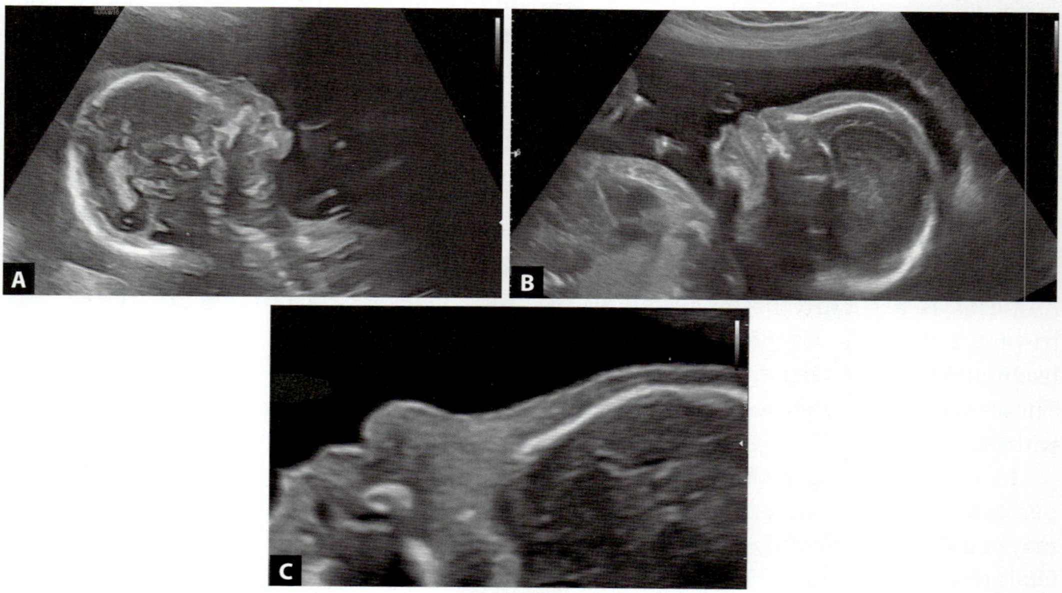

Figs. 10A to C: Abnormal facial profiles in trisomy 21 cases.

trisomy 21 and 0.3–0.7% euploid fetuses. It is hypoplastic in approximately 50–60% fetuses with trisomy 21 and 6–7% euploid fetuses.

Those with negative cell-free DNA screening results and isolated absent or hypoplastic nasal bone, the Society for Maternal-Fetal Medicine (SMFM) recommend further invasive testing depending on clinical circumstances and patient preference.[9]

Mild-to-Moderate Ventriculomegaly (Figs. 11A to C)

Criteria

Ventriculomegaly is identified on a transventricular view of the fetal head. An atrium is measured at the level of the parieto-occipital sulcus with the calipers on the internal margin of the medial and lateral walls of the ventricle. Ventriculomegaly is diagnosed when the atrial diameter is ≥10 mm (irrespective of gestational age), which is 2.5–4 standard deviations above the mean.

Classified as: Mild: 10–12 mm; Moderate: 13–15 mm; or Severe: >15 mm.

Significance

The risk of an abnormal outcome in fetuses with mild ventriculomegaly depends on the cause [e.g., trisomy 21, infection (e.g., cytomegalovirus, toxoplasmosis), and idiopathic] and increases with the degree of ventriculomegaly, progression over time, and presence of other anomalies. Mild-to-moderate ventriculomegaly is detected in 4–13% fetuses with trisomy 21 and 0.1–0.4% euploid fetuses.[8]

Amniocentesis for microarray on amniocytes may be indicated.

Second-trimester Growth Restriction

Criteria

Sonographic estimation of either fetal weight <10th percentile for gestational age or

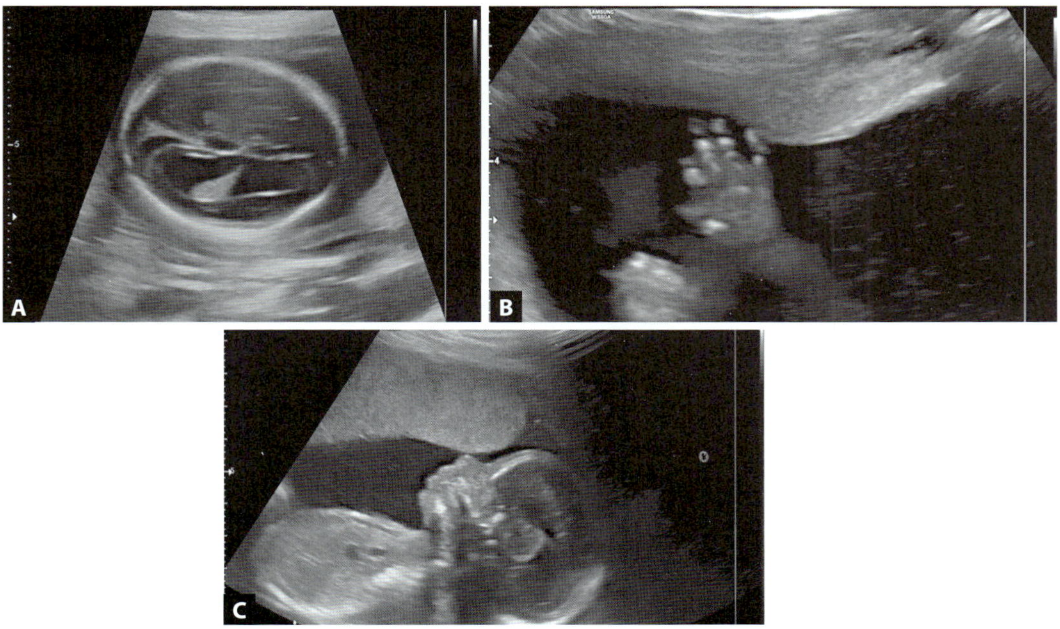

Figs. 11A to C: Case of trisomy 21 with prominent lateral and third ventricle in and other soft markers.

abdominal circumference <10th percentile for gestational age is the popular finding on which to base the diagnosis of FGR.

Significance

Although the most common etiologies for small fetal size are uteroplacental insufficiency and constitutional factors, aneuploidy has been detected in 20% of pregnancies referred for further evaluation of a small fetus. Most growth-restricted fetuses with chromosomal anomalies have associated findings; however, 2–6% of fetuses with isolated growth restriction have an abnormal karyotype. Chromosomal microarray increases the detection of chromosomal abnormalities by 4% in nonanomalous fetuses and by 10% in those with structural abnormalities.

The incidence of growth restriction also varies with the type of aneuploidy. Among fetuses with trisomy 21, 13, and 18, growth restriction has been reported in 30%, 50%, and 90% of cases, respectively.

Suggest a detailed obstetrical ultrasound evaluation, genetic counseling, and offering diagnostic testing for patients with unexplained growth restriction before 32 weeks or anytime in gestation when noted in combination with a fetal malformation or polyhydramnios.[10]

OTHER FINDINGS

- Although more prevalent in fetuses with trisomy 21 than euploid fetuses, markers, such as a sandal gap, short ear length, and a hypoplastic wedge-shaped middle phalanx of the fifth digit that causes it to curve toward the fourth finger (clinodactyly) are common normal variants and are not practically useful for aneuploidy screening.
- An aberrant right subclavian artery **(Figs. 12A and B)** is more common in fetuses with trisomy 21, being seen in 19–28% compared with 1% of euploid fetuses. In fetuses with trisomy 21, it is typically not an isolated finding. It is also not usually associated with cardiac anomalies.[11]

Structural Anomalies

The frequency of chromosomal abnormalities is increased in fetuses with sonographic evidence of structural anomalies. The magnitude of risk for a chromosomal abnormality is highly dependent upon both the specific malformation and the number of malformations.

A low-risk result on cell-free DNA screening may be falsely reassuring in the setting of a structural anomaly.

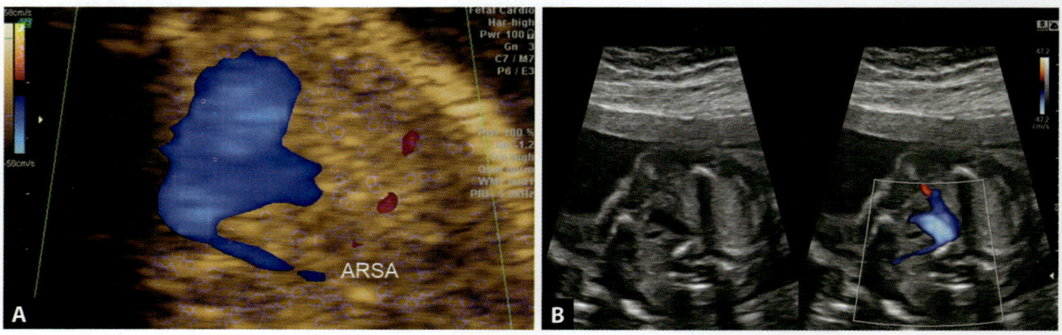

Figs. 12A and B: Aberrant right subclavian artery (ARSA).

REFERENCES

1. American College of Obstetricians and Gynecologists' Committee on Practice Bulletins—Obstetrics, Committee on Genetics, Society for Maternal-Fetal Medicine. Screening for Fetal Chromosomal Abnormalities: ACOG Practice Bulletin, Number 226. Obstet Gynecol. 2020;136(4):e48-69.
2. Bardi F, Bosschieter P, Verheij J, Go A, Haak M, Bekker M, et al. Is there still a role for nuchal translucency measurement in the changing paradigm of first trimester screening? Prenat Diagn. 2020;40:197.
3. Ramkrishna J, Menezes M, Humnabadkar K, Tse C, Maxfield MJ, da Silva Costa F, et al. Outcomes following the detection of fetal edema in early pregnancy prior to non-invasive prenatal testing. Prenat Diagn. 2021;41:241.
4. Schreurs L, Lannoo L, De Catte L, Schoubroeck DV, Devriendt K, Richter J. First trimester cystic hygroma colli: Retrospective analysis in a tertiary center. Eur J Obstet Gynecol Reprod Biol. 2018;231:60.
5. Nicolaides KH. Screening for fetal aneuploidies at 11 to 13 weeks. Prenat Diagn. 2011;31:7.
6. Kao C, Lauzon J, Brundler MA, Tang S, Somerset D. Perinatal outcome and prognostic factors of fetal megacystis diagnosed at 11-14 weeks' gestation. Prenat Diagn. 2021;41:308.
7. Sagi-Dain L, Peleg A, Sagi S. First-trimester crown-rump length and risk of chromosomal aberrations: a systematic review and meta-analysis. Obstet Gynecol Surv. 2017;72:603.
8. Agathokleous M, Chaveeva P, Poon LC, Kosinski P, Nicolaides KH. Meta-analysis of second-trimester markers for trisomy 21. Ultrasound Obstet Gynecol. 2013;41:247.
9. Moreno-Cid M, Rubio-Lorente A, Rodríguez MJ, Pacheco-Bueno G, Tenias JM, Ortiz-Roman C. Systematic review and meta-analysis of performance of second-trimester nasal bone assessment in detection of fetuses with Down syndrome. Ultrasound Obstet Gynecol. 2014;43:247.
10. Society for Maternal-Fetal Medicine (SMFM). Electronic address: pubs@smfm.org; Martins JG, Biggio JR, Abuhamad A. Society for Maternal-Fetal Medicine Consult Series #52: Diagnosis and management of fetal growth restriction: (Replaces Clinical Guideline Number 3, April 2012). Am J Obstet Gynecol. 2020;223:B2.
11. Martínez-Payo C, Suanzes E, Nieto-Jiménez Y, Azúa MR de, Siles A, Usano AI, et al. Is it useful to evaluate the presence of aberrant right subclavian artery in prenatal diagnosis ultrasounds? J Obstet Gynaecol Res. 2021; 47: 359.

7

CHAPTER

Genetic Counseling and Pedigree

Seema Thakur, Preeti Paliwal

KEY POINTS

1. Genetic counseling is a process of communicating medical facts about a genetic disorder.
2. Vast majority of genetic disorders (>90%) would happen to low-risk women without family history, which can be identified by certain blood tests or ultrasound during pregnancy.
3. In the high-risk family seeking prenatal diagnosis, correct etiological diagnosis in the proband is the most critical step for correct prenatal diagnosis and accurate genetic counseling.
4. History taking and examinations along with various investigations both genetic and nongenetic are essential for this.
5. Genetic investigations such as chromosomal microarray, karyotype, and exome sequencing are advised to diagnose the genetic disorder.
6. Once diagnosis is done, family should be provided with most updated information including prognosis, treatment, and recurrence risk.

INTRODUCTION

Over the past few decades, there have been significant advancements in medical genetics, leading to a greater understanding of genetic diseases and testing. The information obtained from genetic testing is particularly valuable in carrier detection, prenatal diagnosis, and postnatal diagnosis, which necessitates the incorporation of these into the clinical practice. The process of assessing individuals and families for the risk and helping them comprehend the medical, psychological, and familial effects as well as the available preventive measures for a genetic disorder is known as genetic counseling. The American Society of Human Genetics defined genetic counseling in 1975 as a communicative process that addresses the human issues associated with the occurrence and/or recurrence of a genetic disorder within a family. An individual seeking genetic counseling is referred to as a consultand.

In the obstetric and gynecologic practice, the indications for genetic counseling continue to evolve as ultrasound and genetic technologies advance. Genetic testing is necessary at various stages for both pregnant and nonpregnant women, including preconception genetic testing, antenatal genetic testing, preimplantation genetic testing (PGT), genetic analysis following fetal demise or fetal malformations, and genetic testing for hereditary cancers. To ensure accurate and effective genetic counseling, the genetic counselor should possess adequate knowledge of obstetrics, radiology, developmental biology, available prenatal as well as postnatal tests/procedures, and genetics.

Common reasons for referral to genetic counseling in pregnancy and preconception period include both low- and high-risk women. Low-risk women have abnormalities detected during pregnancy and high-risk women are those who already have a personal/family history of genetic disorder.

LOW-RISK WOMEN

- Positive screening test such as double marker
- Advanced maternal age
- Advanced paternal age
- Nuchal translucency (NT) >95th centile
- Soft markers on ultrasound
- Fetal anomalies on ultrasound
- Exposure to certain teratogenic drugs during pregnancy, e.g., valproate, isotretinoin
- Abnormal high-performance liquid chromatography (HPLC) results
- Prenatal diagnosis for Down syndrome or other chromosomal/copy number variation (CNV) abnormalities
- Prenatal diagnosis for thalassemia or other single-gene disorders
- Noninvasive prenatal screening (NIPS)
- Abnormal NIPS
- Abnormal chromosomal microarray reports
- Abnormal whole exome sequencing results
- Expanded carrier screening

HIGH-RISK WOMEN

- Previous child with intellectual disability, autism, or a genetic disorder
- Family history of genetic disorders or breast/ovarian cancer
- Balanced translocation carrier in couple
- Recurrent abortions
- Primary amenorrhea
- Infertility

STEPS OF GENETIC COUNSELING

1. Diagnosis by medical history, family history, examination, investigations, and pedigree drawing
2. Risk assessment
3. Communication
4. Discussion of reproductive options

Basically, the entire counseling process is divided into pretest genetic counseling and post-test genetic counseling. Pretest genetic counseling is for making a clinical diagnosis and genetic testing. Post-test counseling is about interpretation of genetic reports and clinical correlation including discussion of medical aspects of the genetic disorder. Post-test counseling also involves recurrence risk counseling.

An important component of genetic counseling is nondirectiveness. Nondirective counseling is an approach that presents factual information without influencing the couple's decision-making process. The counselor should provide the couple with all available information about the disease and reproductive options, allowing them to make their own decisions. It is essential to maintain a nondirective stance throughout the counseling process.

Pretest Genetic Counseling

- Etiological diagnosis through medical history, family history, pedigree drawing, physical examination, and relevant investigations
- Genetic testing of proband. If proband is not available, parental testing is done
- Cost, benefits, and limitations of the testing including a discussion on the false positives and false negatives, variants of uncertain significance, and turnaround time
- Implications of the genetic testing.

Post-test Genetic Counseling

- Interpretation of the test result and clinical correlation including testing of parents/ other family members
- Counseling regarding prognosis including treatment
- Counseling regarding recurrence risk
- Discussion of available reproductive options.

The genetic counseling typically starts from history taking and drawing a three-generation pedigree, which involves gathering information on the family and drawing a family tree which is a shorthand system of recording the pertinent information about a family. Pedigree chart typically outlines the relationships among family members and their affected or unaffected status for a specific trait or disorder. It usually begins with the person through whom the family came to the attention of the investigator. This person is referred to as the index case or proband and is indicated by an arrow. Information about the health of the rest of the family is obtained by asking direct questions about brothers, sisters, parents, and the relatives of parents (maternal/paternal). This information is then used for interpretation of the inheritance patterns of traits or disorders within a family across multiple generations.

Pedigree analysis is valuable in determining the mode of inheritance [autosomal dominant (AD), autosomal recessive (AR), X-linked, etc.] of a trait or disorder, estimating the risk of recurrence in future generations, identifying carriers, and understanding the underlying genetic mechanisms.

Pedigree symbols are graphic representations used in genetics to depict relationships and inheritance patterns within a family. Some commonly used pedigree symbols are as follows **(Fig. 1)**:

Square (male): A square is used to represent a male individual in a pedigree. It is typically placed on the left side.

Circle (female): A circle is used to represent a female individual in a pedigree. It is usually placed on the right side.

Diamond (unknown gender): A diamond is used to represent an individual whose gender is unknown or undisclosed.

Filled-in shape: When a square, circle, or diamond is completely filled in, it indicates that the individual has the specific trait or condition being studied.

Line (marriage/partnership): A horizontal line connects a male and female symbol to represent a marriage or partnership.

Vertical line (parent–child relationship): A vertical line connecting a male or female symbol to a child symbol indicates a parent–child relationship.

Siblings: Sibling relationships are depicted by horizontal lines that connect children born to the same parents. These lines connect the lower portion of the symbols representing the siblings.

Generations: Different generations are represented by placing symbols in different rows, with each row corresponding to a different generation.

Roman numerals: Roman numerals (I, II, III, etc.) are often used above the symbols to label different generations.

These symbols are used to construct a pedigree chart or diagram that provides a visual representation of familial relationships, inheritance patterns, and the occurrence of specific traits or conditions within a family.

Some key steps involved in pedigree analysis are as follows:

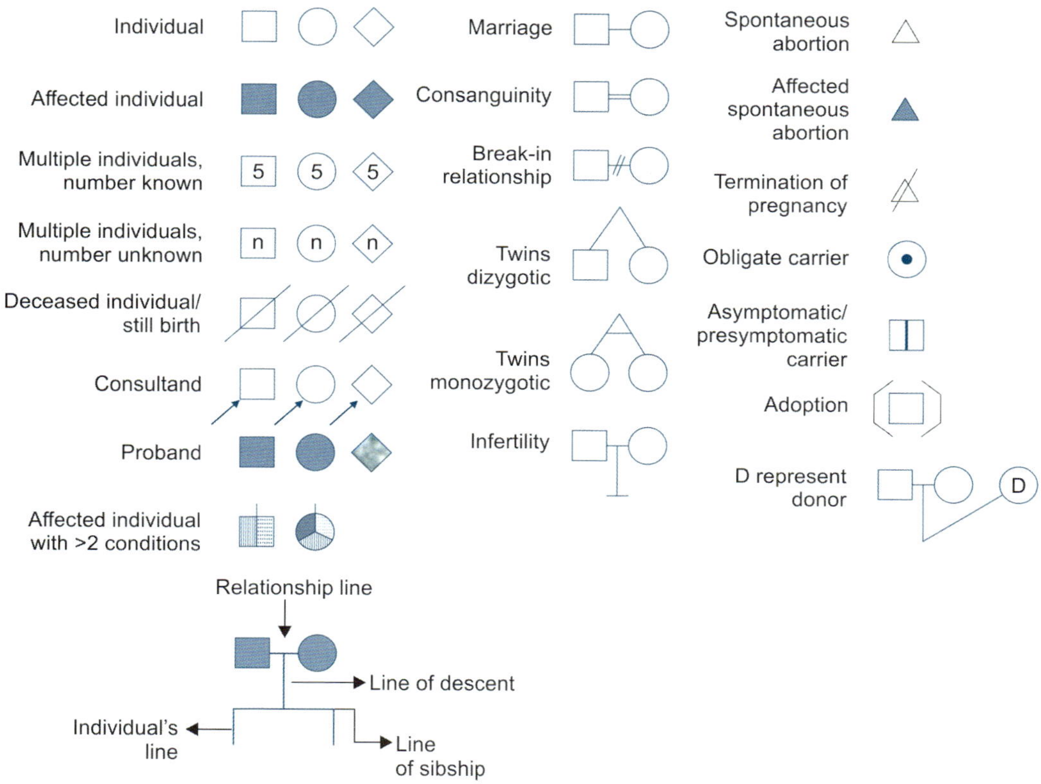

Fig. 1

Collecting information: A detailed information about the trait or disorder of interest from multiple generations of the family is gathered. This includes obtaining medical records, conducting interviews with family members, and documenting the presence or absence of the trait or disorder.

Constructing the pedigree chart: A pedigree chart or family tree using standard symbols to represent individuals, their gender, relationships, and affected or unaffected status is constructed. Typically, squares represent males, circles represent females, shaded symbols represent affected individuals, and half-shaded symbols represent carriers.

Analyzing inheritance patterns: The pedigree is examined for the patterns of inheritance such as the presence or absence of the trait or disorder in each generation, the sex of affected individuals, and whether the trait or disorder is passed from parent to offspring.

Determining the mode of inheritance: Based on the observed patterns, determine the most likely mode of inheritance (AD, AR, X-linked, etc.).

Inheritance patterns can be classified into Mendelian inheritance and non-Mendelian inheritance. Mendelian inheritance refers to the inheritance of traits or disorders that are caused by single genes. It includes AD inheritance, AR inheritance, X-linked recessive inheritance, and X-linked dominant inheritance. Non-Mendelian disorders include triplet repeat disorders, imprinting disorders, etc.

Autosomal dominant inheritance occurs when a single copy of an abnormal gene is sufficient to cause the disease. Both males and females can be affected, and the disorder can be passed on to the next generation. Some examples of AD disorders are achondroplasia, osteogenesis imperfecta, and Marfan syndrome. The risk of transmitting the disorder to the next generation is 50% for affected individuals. AD disorders can also occur sporadically for the first time in a family, in which case the risk of recurrence is around 6% due to gonadal mosaicism **(Fig. 2)**.

Autosomal recessive inheritance occurs when both copies of a gene contain pathogenic variants. Both males and females can be affected, and the parents are usually carriers of the abnormal gene. The risk of occurrence/recurrence in each pregnancy for an affected child is 25%. Thalassemia, spinal muscular atrophy, and cystic fibrosis are examples of AR disorders **(Fig. 3)**.

X-linked recessive inheritance primarily affects males because they have only one copy of the X chromosome. Carrier females can pass on the gene to their sons, who may be affected, while their daughters have a 50% chance of being carriers. Examples of X-linked recessive disorders are color blindness, hemophilia A, and Duchenne muscular dystrophy **(Fig. 4)**.

X-linked dominant inheritance manifests in both heterozygous females and affected males. The gene can be passed on by affected females to their offspring, with a 50% chance of transmission in each pregnancy; however, there is no male-to-male transmission. Examples include vitamin D-resistant rickets and incontinentia pigmenti.

In addition to Mendelian inheritance, there are non-Mendelian patterns of inheritance as mentioned below:

- Triple repeat disorders are expansions of repeated sequences of three nucleotides,

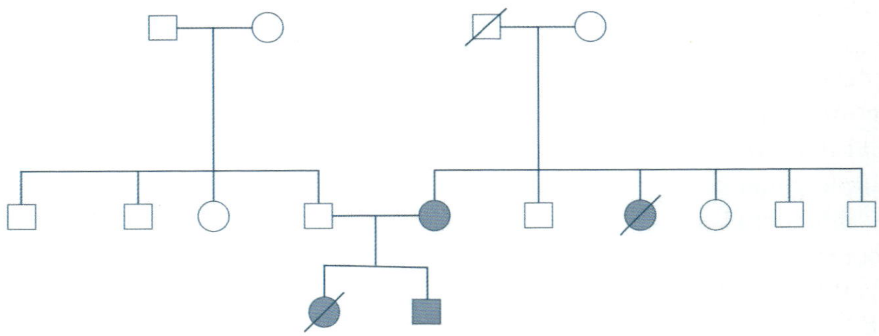

Fig. 2: Autosomal dominant pedigree in a case of Li–Fraumeni syndrome caused by *P53* gene pathogenic variant.

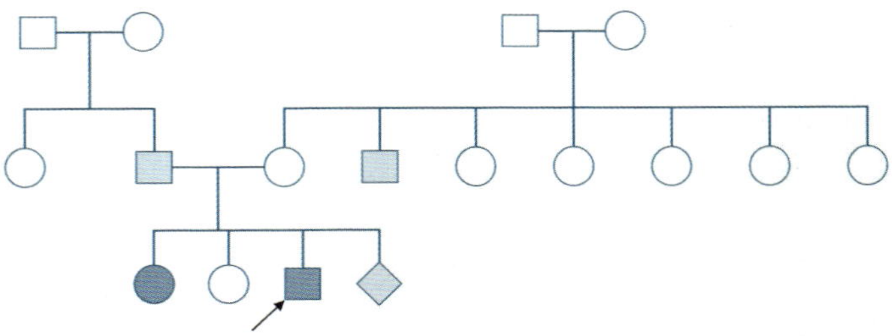

Fig. 3: Autosomal recessive pedigree in a case of thalassemia major in two siblings.

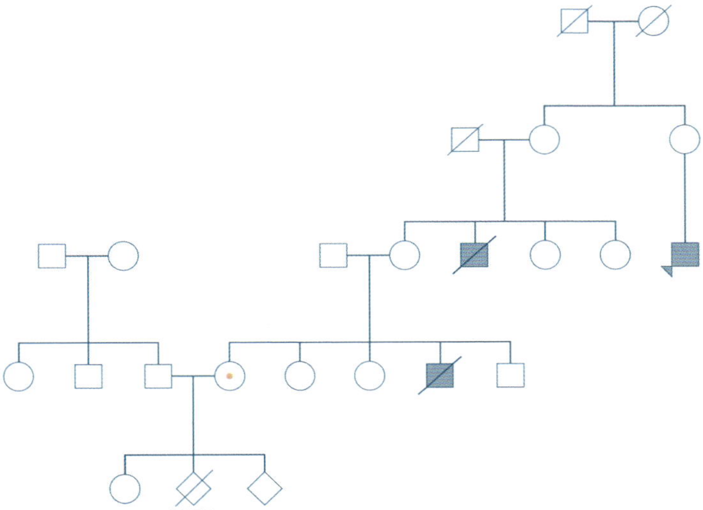

Fig. 4: X-linked recessive pedigree in a case of hemophilia in two generations.

which can lead to diseases such as fragile X syndrome, Huntington's chorea, and myotonic dystrophy.

- Imprinting is a process in which the expression of certain genes varies based on the sex of the parent from whom they were inherited. Examples of imprinting disorders are Angelman syndrome and Prader–Willi syndrome.
- Uniparental disomy (UPD) occurs when both sets of a chromosome pair are inherited from one parent, which can lead to imprinting disorders.
- Mitochondrial inheritance involves the inheritance of traits encoded in the mitochondrial genome and is passed down maternally or can be inherited as AR if mutation occurs in nuclear genes controlling mitochondrial genome.

Understanding the inheritance patterns and their implications is essential in genetic counseling and providing accurate recurrence risks to individuals and families.

Autosomal dominant disorders often appear in every successive generation, affecting both males and females. AR disorders generally affect one generation, both males and females, and often have unaffected carrier parents. X-linked disorders primarily affect males and are passed from carrier females to their sons and affect more than one generation like AD inheritance. The major difference between AD and X-linked disorder is that in X-linked disorders, there is no male-to-male transmission.

CALCULATING RECURRENCE RISKS

Once the mode of inheritance (single-gene disorders) is determined, the risk of recurrence is calculated for future offspring. AD disorders have a 50% chance of being passed on by an affected parent. AR disorders have a 25% chance of occurring in offspring when both parents are carriers. In X-linked recessive disorders, 50% of males are affected and 50% of females are carriers.

However, chromosome disorders have different recurrence risks. For example, as in the case of Down syndrome, the recurrence risk depends on the karyotype of the index case. The recurrence risk for the next child is 1% above the background risk for previous trisomy 21. Translocation type of Down syndrome can be de novo or inherited from parents. In the case of an inherited translocation from parents, the risk varies from 5 to 30%, depending on the type of translocation.

The results are then communicated by genetic counselors, clinical geneticists, or other healthcare professionals with expertise in genetics.

COMMUNICATION

- After establishing a diagnosis, it should be communicated to the patient and family.
- Preferably face-to-face communication in a quiet and isolated room should be performed. Online genetic counseling can be an alternative if the patient prefers it.
- Ideally, both partners should be present during the counseling session.
- The genetic counselor should be an empathetic listener and must use simple language to convey clear messages.
- Pictures/charts should be used to simplify explanations of genetic testing.
- The counseling session should cover all aspects of the disease, including etiology, diagnosis, treatment, course, prognosis, and recurrence risk.

REPRODUCTIVE OPTIONS

Once the risk of recurrence has been discussed, various reproductive options should be presented to the couple, including:

- Prenatal diagnosis through chorionic villus sampling (CVS) or amniocentesis
- In vitro fertilization (IVF) with PGT
- IVF with donor oocyte or sperm
- Adoption

During the counseling session, it is important to discuss the accuracy and limitations of prenatal diagnostic tests, the risks associated with invasive testing, and the considerations related to termination of pregnancy and permitted time limit as per the law should be discussed. Additionally, the counselor should provide up-to-date information about the disease and the availability of the centers for facilities for prenatal diagnosis.

SUGGESTED READING

1. Phadke S. Handbook of Genetic Counselling.
2. Turnpenny PD, Ellard S. Emery's Elements of Medical Genetics. Philadelphia: Elsevier; 2017.

Quiz 1

Jaya Chawla

1. Preconceptional folate 4 mg a day is advisable to:
   a. All women of reproductive age
   b. Women with history of neural tube defects
   c. Women on anticonvulsant drugs
   d. Women with a history of cardiac defects such as tetralogy of Fallot
2. A primigravida women presents to the antenatal care with an ultrasound showing abdominal circumference <3rd centile at 30 weeks. She has no comorbid conditions. What substance abuse could be associated with her condition?
   a. Cocaine b. Tobacco
   c. Marijuana d. Opioids
3. A 36-year-old G2P1L1 patient who initially presented with pregnancy of unknown location was diagnosed with right-sided tubal ectopic pregnancy at 7-week gestation and administered conservative management and discharged. She presents at 20 weeks with an anomaly scan suggestive of micrognathia bilateral club feet and bilateral choroid plexus cysts (CPCs) 0.5 cm each. The radiologist has expressed some concern over the shape of the skull as well. What condition/teratogen could be associated with this presentation?
   a. Trisomy 21 b. Mifepristone
   c. Misoprostol d. Methotrexate
4. A 24-year-old retrovirus positive primigravida presents to the antenatal clinic with a second trimester anomaly scan suggestive of stippled epiphysis. She delivers a baby at term with scaphocephaly as shown in the figure. What therapeutic agents could most likely be associated with this outcome?

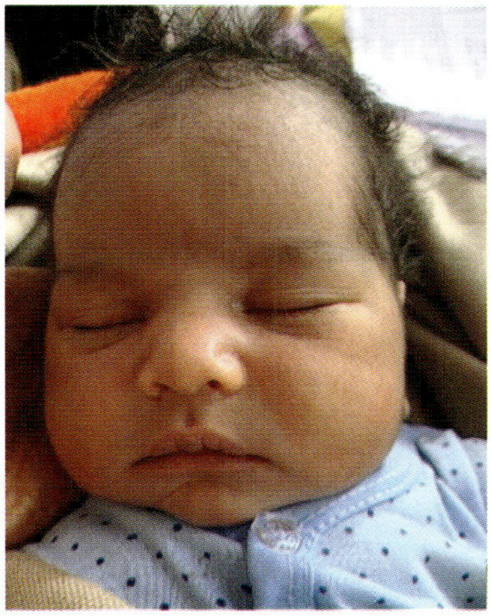

   a. Antibacterial drugs
   b. Antiviral drugs
   c. Antiretroviral drugs
   d. Antifungal drugs
5. The recommended threshold for optimization of overt diabetes mellitus in periconceptional period as per the American Diabetes Association is:
   a. <6% b. <6.3%
   c. <7% d. <7.3%
6. A couple presents for post-test counseling following noninvasive prenatal screening (NIPS) requested for

an intermediate risk result for trisomy 21 obtained on combined first-trimester screening (CFTS). The result is low risk. However, this does not completely absolve them of the possibility of a baby with Down syndrome. What is this concept known as?

a. Negative likelihood ratio (NLR)
b. Negative predictive value (NPV)
c. Residual risk
d. A priori risk

7. A 32-year-old lady presents to the outpatient department (OPD) at 15 weeks' gestation with a combined risk report suggestive of high risk of trisomy 21 on CFTS. On further scrutiny, she is found to have pregnancy-associated plasma protein-A (PAPP-A) 0.8 multiples of median (MoM), free beta human chorionic gonadotropin (BhCG) 1.3 MoM, crown rump length (CRL) = 76 mm; nuchal translucency (NT) 3.8 mm; no tricuspid regurgitation (TR), and positive "a" wave on ductus venosus (DV) Doppler. What would be the best possible counseling for her in the light of current evidence?
   a. Invasive testing
   b. NIPS
   c. Quadruple marker
   d. No further testing until midtrimester anomaly scan

8. A 32-year-old lady presents to the OPD at 24 weeks' gestation with a low-risk report on NIPS following a high-risk CFTS. She had PAPP-A 0.3 MoM, free BhCG 1.3 MoM, CRL = 76 mm; NT 1.8 mm; no TR, and positive "a" wave on DV Doppler. How would she be counseled for her ongoing pregnancy?
   a. She should be offered screening for gestational diabetes mellitus (GDM)
   b. She should be offered surveillance for preeclampsia (PE) and fetal growth restriction (FGR)
   c. She should be offered routine antenatal care since she is low risk on NIPS
   d. She should be offered a fetal echo given her high risk on CFTS

9. A 32-year-old lady presents to the OPD at 24 weeks' gestation with a normal karyotype report following a high-risk CFTS. She had PAPP-A 0.8 MoM, free BhCG 1.3 MoM, CRL = 76 mm; NT 3.8 mm; no TR, and positive "a" wave on DV Doppler. How should she be counseled for her ongoing pregnancy?
   a. Routine antenatal care
   b. Risk of intrauterine fetal demise 2%
   c. Surveillance for early onset PE/FGR
   d. Fetal echo

10. A 32-year-old lady G2P1L1 with a previous baby with Down syndrome presents to the OPD at 17 weeks' gestation with a combined risk report suggestive of high risk of trisomy 21 on CFTS. On further scrutiny, her CFTS is found to have PAPP-A 0.8 MoM, free BhCG 1.3 MoM, CRL = 76 mm; NT 2.7 mm; absent nasal bone; no TR, and positive "a" wave on DV Doppler. Her repeat scan continues to show absent nasal bone. So, the couple opt for invasive testing. What tests should be requested on the amniotic fluid sample?
    a. Fluorescence in situ hybridization (FISH) followed by chromosome microarray analysis (CMA) if former is normal
    b. FISH followed by CMA, if former is abnormal
    c. Karyotype
    d. Quantitative fluorescent polymerase chain reaction (QF PCR)

11. With an algorithmic approach utilizing maternal high-risk factors with mean arterial pressure (MAP), mean uterine artery pulsatility index (PI) and serum markers, what is the cutoff to label a patient as high risk?
    a. 1:250 b. 1: 1,000
    c. 1:100 d. 1: 200
12. The *gestosis score* is useful tool in the low-resource setting to identify women at risk of developing PE. Which of the following combinations shall have the highest score?
    a. Age <19 years/pregnancy with surrogacy/primigravida
    b. History of polycystic ovarian disease (PCOD)/in vitro fertilization (IVF) conception/multiple pregnancy
    c. History of mental disorder/hypothyroidism/anemia
    d. Systemic lupus erythematosus (SLE)/age >35 years/MAP >85 mm Hg
13. A 32-year-old G3P2L2 woman with 32 weeks' pregnancy has brought her biomarker report for assessment of risk for late-onset PE. Which of the following would be suggestive of high risk?
    a. Increased soluble fms-like tyrosine kinase-1 (sFLT-1) and placental growth factor (PlGF)
    b. Decreased sFLT-1 and decreased PlGF
    c. Increased sFLT-1 decreased PlGF
    d. Decreased sFLT-1 increased PlGF
14. A 38-year-old G2P1L1 woman presents at 22 weeks' gestation with history of PE with severe features in a previous pregnancy. She is currently normotensive. Which of the following will not help to improve her risk assessment over and above maternal factors for the development of preeclampsia?
    a. Uterine artery PI
    b. MAP
    c. PlGF
    d. sFLT-1
15. Which of the following biomarkers has the best performance in the diagnosis and subsequent triaging of patients with PE in first trimester?
    a. sFLT-1
    b. PlGF
    c. Glycosylated fibronectin
    d. PAPP-A
16. In order to optimize resolution for fetal spine, one should:
    a. Use a lower frequency transducer, say 2–5 MHz
    b. Use a higher frequency transducer, say 5–12 MHz
    c. Place the focal zone in the region of the spine or anterior to it
    d. Turn off tissue harmonic imaging
17. The thermal index is a measure of the potential for thermal tissue damage attributable to ultrasound. Which of the following are true about thermal index?
    a. It is expressed as a risk, say 1:250
    b. It is independent of power and frequency of ultrasound waves
    c. Thermal index is different for different tissues
    d. The risk to the fetus is inversely proportional to the thermal index
18. While imaging dynamic structures, such as the fetal heart, one must do all, *except*:
    a. Keeping the frame rate low
    b. Keeping the sector width narrow
    c. Decreasing depth
    d. Using color map
19. The following are true for gain:
    a. One must enhance gain to see the echogenic cardiac foci clearly
    b. Gain must be enhanced to clearly visualize the NT endpoints
    c. It is crucial to lower gain to appropriately appreciate echogenic bowel
    d. Gain must be adjusted such that the urinary bladder appears echo free

20. The following hold true for the zoom/depth function:
    a. Write zoom improves image resolution
    b. Read zoom improves image resolution
    c. Increasing depth leads to increase in frame rates
    d. Increasing depth leads to better resolution
21. For the measurement of head circumference (HC), the following hold true:
    a. Ellipse should be placed on the outer edge of the calvarium
    b. Ellipse should be placed on the inner edge of the calvarium
    c. Ellipse function is superior to HC computed using biparietal diameter (BPD) and occipitofrontal diameter (OFD)
    d. Ellipse function is inferior to HC computed using BPD and OFD
22. Why is PI the preferred index to be incorporated in obstetric imaging?
    a. It incorporates average values rather than maximum/minimum points
    b. It reaches infinity with absent or reversed flows
    c. Resistance index (RI) is superior to PI for obstetric measurements
    d. Peak systolic velocity better reflects fetal hemodynamics
23. Cerebroplacental ratio (CPR) is the criteria for:
    a. Early-onset FGR
    b. Encephalocele
    c. Late-onset FGR
    d. Placental mesenchymal dysplasia
24. With respect to middle cerebral artery (MCA):
    a. Umbilical artery/MCA peak systolic velocity = CPR
    b. Fetal MCA peak systolic velocity is related to rheological properties of maternal blood
    c. MCA PI <5th centile is a marker of fetal compromise that sets in earlier than the deterioration of CPR
    d. To locate the MCA, one should identify the base of skull view
25. Reversed end-diastolic flow in the umbilical artery at 30 weeks' gestation should be followed by:
    a. Immediate termination of pregnancy
    b. DV PI evaluation
    c. CPR evaluation
    d. MAP PI evaluation
26. A 32-year-old lady comes to the antenatal OPD at 22 weeks' gestation with a normal karyotype report for amniocentesis done for raised NT >99%. What are the important aspects to be covered in her post-test counseling?
    a. No further testing as aneuploidy has been ruled out
    b. Fetal echo because her NT was raised
    c. Deoxyribonucleic acid (DNA) stored as she may have RASopathies such as Noonan's syndrome
    d. Quadruple marker
27. A 24-year-old primigravida comes for first-trimester scan as part of combined screen. CRL 76 mm; NT 1.9 mm; no TR; DV shows positive "a" wave; absent nasal bone at 13 weeks and 4 days. Counseling must include all of the following, *except*:
    a. Invasive testing to rule out aneuploidy
    b. Invasive testing followed by microarray
    c. Review scan at 16–17 weeks
    d. Quadruple marker

28. Most common association of CPC is with:
    a. Trisomy 13
    b. Trisomy 18
    c. Trisomy 21
    d. Turner's syndrome
29. Reversed "a" wave on DV Doppler. All of the following are true, *except*:
    a. The baby may have an aneuploidy
    b. Fetal echo must be offered to rule out cardiac abnormalities
    c. Majority of babies with the finding shall be normal
    d. There remains a risk of intrauterine fetal demise despite aneuploidy being ruled out
30. When echogenic bowel is seen on a second-trimester scan, all of the following must be ruled out, *except*:
    a. Cystic fibrosis
    b. Congenital infection
    c. Intra-amniotic bleeding
    d. FGR

ANSWERS

1. b, c	2. a, b, d	3. d	4. d	5. c
6. c	7. a	8. b	9. d	10. a
11. c	12. c	13. c	14. d	15. b
16. a/d	17. c	18. a	19. c, d	20. a
21. a/c	22. a	23. c	24. d	25. b
26. b/c	27. d	28. b	29. c	30. None of the above

CHAPTER 8

Genetic Testing: Which and When

Ratna Dua Puri, Veronica Arora, Meena Lall, Sudha Kohli, Sudhisha Dubey

KEY POINTS

1. Genetic testing in obstetrics plays a pivotal role in prenatal care, offering insights into the genetic makeup of the fetus, thus aiding in the detection of chromosomal abnormalities and genetic disorders.
2. Fluorescence in situ hybridization (FISH) provides a quick turnaround but is limited by the need to know which specific abnormality to test for.
3. Karyotyping offers a broader view by examining the entire chromosome set for structural or numerical changes.
4. Chromosomal microarray analysis (CMA) has become a standard for identifying chromosomal imbalances at a higher resolution than karyotyping.
5. Indicated for individuals with developmental delays, congenital anomalies, or abnormal fetal ultrasound findings, CMA can detect copy number variations (CNVs) not visible on karyotype.
6. Multiplex ligation-dependent probe amplification (MLPA) is a technique used to detect copy number changes in specific genomic regions. It is particularly useful for conditions caused by deletions or duplications of small segments, such as certain hereditary cancer syndromes, Duchene muscular dystrophy, spinal muscular atrophy.
7. Sanger sequencing, the gold standard for precise genetic mutation identification, is utilized for the detection of single-gene disorders.
8. Exome sequencing (ES) examines the coding regions of genes (exome), where most known genetic variant mutations are found. Indicated for complex cases with suspected genetic disorders where other tests have failed to provide a diagnosis, it offers a comprehensive solution.
9. In prenatal ES a thorough knowledge is required for interpreting the variant of unknown significance.
10. The choice of test depends on the clinical context, with a thorough understanding of each method's capabilities and limitations being crucial for informed decision-making in prenatal care.

INTRODUCTION

The burden of genetic disorders in India is now being realized as the incidence of infectious diseases is decreasing with improved neonatal care facilities. In the absence of robust registry data, estimates of neonatal births with congenital anomalies and genetic disorder varies from 5.3 to 7.9% that translates to 15 lakhs per year.

Over the years, the scope of genetics has increased vastly with the availability of genetic and genomic tests along with enhanced imaging technology. Integration of baseline clinical information, imaging, genomic testing, and appropriate counseling now enables enhanced screening and diagnostic opportunities for prevention of birth defects and genetic disorders. This chapter focuses on the various genetic and genomic technologies and their application in the care of the unborn fetus. With the aid of examples, this primer for medical students and young doctors will focus on the requisite preliminary information that is imperative to decide the appropriate genetic test and the correct interpretation within the scope of fetal medicine practice.

In this chapter, we will address the basics of genetic testing, different types of genetic tests, indications of testing, and advantages and limitations of the tests with case examples.

BASICS OF GENETIC AND GENOMIC TESTING

Within the context of this chapter, this refers to the analysis of the human genome that comprises the nuclear content including chromosomes or the deoxyribonucleic acid (DNA). There are 23 pairs of chromosomes and each chromosome is composed of two chromatids made of condensed DNA strands attached at the centromere. Alternating combinations of the four nucleotides, ACGT (adenine, cytosine, guanine, and thymine), comprise the genes within the DNA strand. There are about 20,000 genes and these comprise only 1–2% of the genome.

TYPES OF GENETIC TESTS

Genetic tests in the practice of fetal genetics can be classified as screening tests and diagnostic tests.

- *Screening tests:* They include serum biomarkers, ultrasonographic soft markers associated with aneuploidy, fetal imaging for growth and malformations, and cell-free fetal DNA (cffDNA) analysis for rhesus (Rh) testing and aneuploidy.
- *Diagnostic tests:* These are confirmatory tests and include:
  - Tests for chromosomal disorders:
    - Fluorescence in situ hybridization
    - Karyotype
    - Chromosomal microarray analysis
  - Tests for monogenic disorders:
    - PCR-based tests
    - DNA sequencing
    - Next-generation sequencing

Screening Tests for Down Syndrome and Other Aneuploidies

The two main components of this screening are: Analysis of specific biomarkers in maternal serum and ultrasound markers to determine the likelihood for trisomy 21, 13, and 18 in the fetus. The risk for neural tube defect is also ascertained with maternal alpha-fetoprotein (AFP) levels.

The first-trimester combined screen is performed between 11 to 13 weeks and 6 days of gestation to assess the risk of trisomy 21, 18, and 13. Serum-free human chorionic gonadotropin [free beta human chorionic gonadotropin (fβ-hCG)] and pregnancy-associated plasma protein-A (PAPP-A) are tested. This test in conjunction with the nuchal translucency (NT) scan has a sensitivity of 85% for trisomy 21.

In the second trimester, screening is performed with the quadruple marker test, performed between 16 to 20 weeks of pregnancy and measures the levels AFP, hCG, estriol, and inhibin A. The test can detect 65–70% of the fetuses with trisomy 21. An added advantage is screening for open neural tube defects by the AFP component of the test. Triple test is not recommended these days for aneuploidy screening due to lower accuracy compared to other available screening tests.

It is important to note that these serum biomarkers are screening tests that can only identify pregnancies at higher risk for chromosomal abnormalities, but they cannot diagnose these conditions with certainty. If the results of these screening tests indicate an increased risk of chromosomal abnormalities, further testing such as chorionic villus sampling (CVS) or amniocentesis should be recommended to provide a definitive diagnosis.

Noninvasive Prenatal Screening

Noninvasive prenatal screening (NIPS) is based on the presence of cffDNA in the maternal blood. This DNA is released from the cytotrophoblasts into the circulation and sequenced to detect chromosome imbalances. The proportion of this DNA is adequate to be tested starting at 9 weeks' gestation and a maternal blood sample can undergo testing any time after this gestation.

Noninvasive prenatal screening is highly accurate screening test with a sensitivity of 98.80% [95% confidence interval (CI) 97.81–99.34] and a specificity of 99.96% (95% CI 99.92–99.98) for trisomy 21 with a false-positive rate of 0.09%. It is an accurate screening test for the common aneuploidies of chromosome 21, 13, and 18. False-positive NIPS are reported and every screen-positive test must be followed by confirmatory diagnostic invasive testing. NIPS will not detect structural anomalies. There are various methods to implement NIPS—primary screen, though not preferred at a primary level in India due to cost, contingent to a prior positive aneuploidy screen. Academic societies confirm NIPS as an efficient screening modality for the above aneuploidies and allow individual decisions on the model to be implemented in countries. Rare autosomal trisomies and subchromosomal imbalances including microdeletions and microduplications testing by NIPS are not recommended.

Pre- and post-test genetic counseling is essential. This is not the test of choice in the presence of fetal structural malformations or increased nuchal translucency.

Rhesus genotyping of fetus by noninvasive testing (cell-free fetal DNA from maternal blood): Rhesus incompatibility occurs in RhD-negative mothers when they carry a RhD-positive fetus. If she is sensitized and produces anti-D antibodies (alloimmunization), these cross the placenta and can cause fetal anemia if the fetus is Rh (D) positive. This is the most common cause of fetal anemia. If the mother is RhD negative and father is RhD positive, there is a one-third chance that the fetus is RhD negative. The actual RhD status of the husband is ascertained by RhD genotyping. If the father is RhD±, then fetal RhD testing is performed in maternal plasma by cffDNA testing. In this situation, noninvasive fetal RhD testing in maternal blood is recommended. The sensitivity of this test is 97.2% and specificity is 96.8%.

If the fetus is RhD negative, no further monitoring is required for fetal anemia. If the fetus is RhD positive, then the pregnancy is followed up by antibody titers and middle cerebral artery (MCA) Doppler assessments as per guidelines. It is essential to do father's RhD genotype before fetal RhD testing.

TESTS FOR CHROMOSOMAL DISORDERS

Karyotype

A *karyotype* examines all 23 pairs of chromosomes. These are visualized under the microscope and arranged according to their G-bands, their descending order of size, and presence of the centromere position. Karyotype will examine the whole genome and identify abnormalities in chromosome number and large (>5–10 Mb) structural abnormalities. The latter include chromosomal deletions, duplications, isochromosomes, inversion, ring chromosomes, extra structural abnormal chromosome (ESACs or markers) and balanced and unbalanced translocations. Their diagnostic accuracy of karyotype in amniotic fluid (AF) and CVS being 99.4–99.8% and 97.5–99.6%, respectively (Shaffer et al., 2007).

Figure 1 depicts an abnormality of chromosomal number where the child has Down syndrome due to an extra chromosome 21.

Figure 2 depicts a structural chromosomal abnormality that is a translocation of genomic material between chromosomes 1 and 13.

Sample for Karyotype

- Peripheral blood in heparin anticoagulant vacutainer
- Chorionic villi or AF sample
- Skin fibroblasts

Indications of Karyotype in Fetal Medicine

- Screen-positive first- or second-trimester aneuploidy screen test
- A parent is a carrier of a balanced translocation.

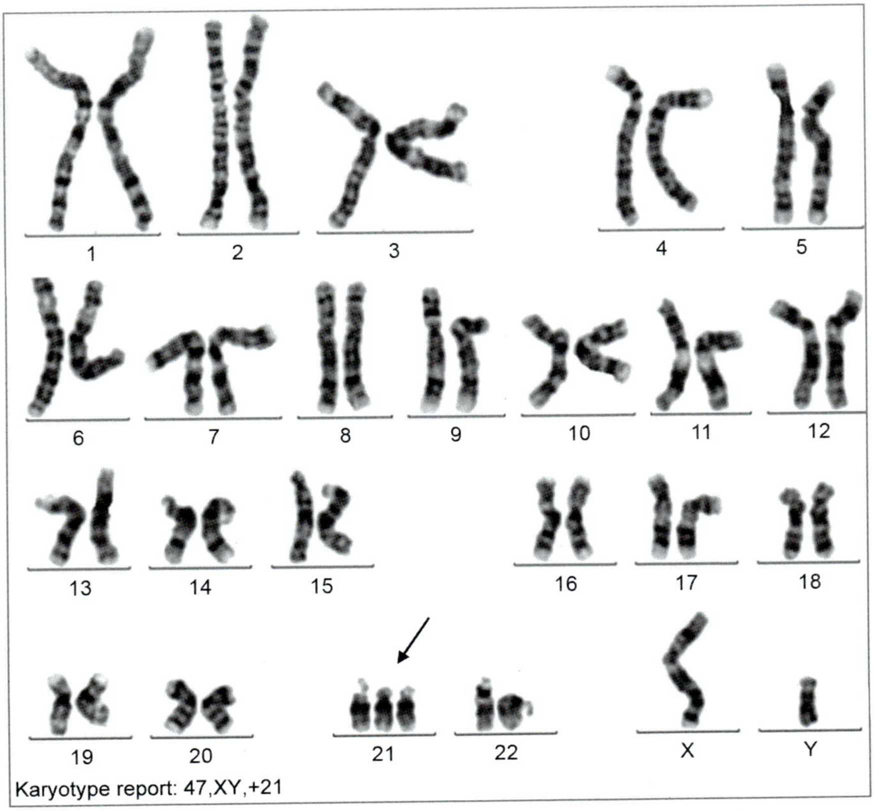

Fig. 1: Karyotype showing a chromosomal abnormality of number.

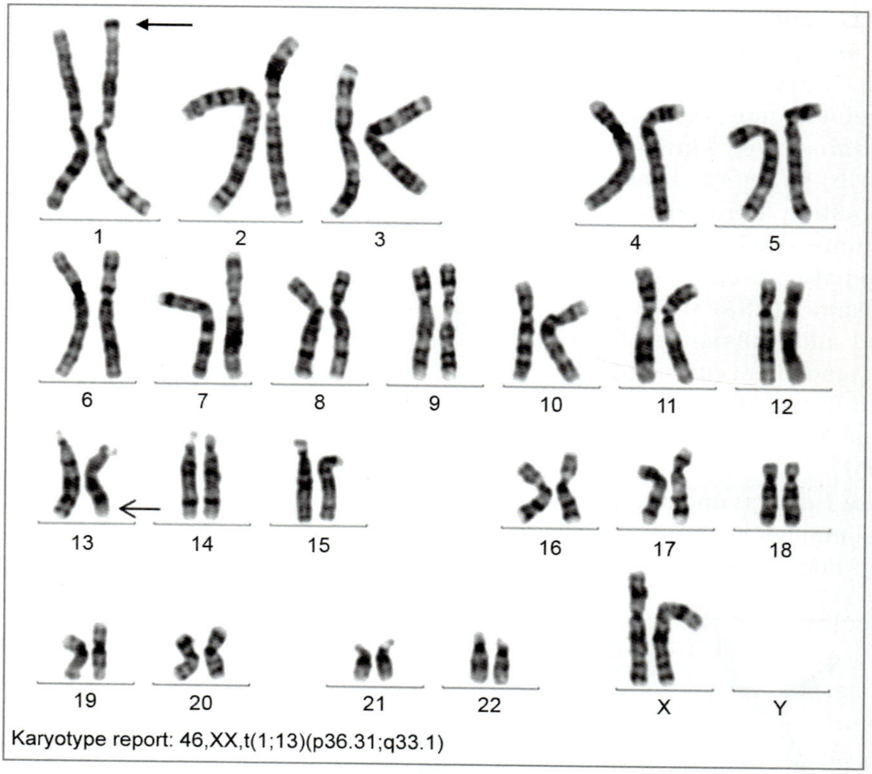

Fig. 2: Karyotype showing a balanced translocation, an abnormality of chromosome structure.

- Fetal malformations suggesting a specific disorder, e.g., duodenal atresia and risk for trisomy 21.
- Fetal malformations when CMA is not possible.
- Confirmation of fetal chromosomes after preimplantation genetic testing for structural rearrangement (PGT-SR).
- Other indications related to obstetric practice include primary amenorrhea, recurrent pregnancy loss, and infertility.

Limitations of Karyotype

Limitations include a resolution up to 5–10 million base pairs. Small deletions and duplications will not be identified by karyotype. Karyotyping requires cultured cells from blood, AF cell, or CVS to arrest dividing or mitotic cells at metaphase when the chromosomes are visible microscopically **(Fig. 3)**.

Fluorescent in situ Hybridization

Fluorescent in situ hybridization is a targeted approach when there is a specific suspicion of a particular chromosomal abnormality based on ultrasound findings or family history. The cells of prenatal samples (AF or CVS) or of the blood sample of the patient are immobilized on the glass slides and hybridized with the now commercially available DNA probes of the targeted genomic region to detect the particular disorder for which probes are used. This can provide rapid results compared to other techniques like karyotyping or CMA. Examples of common FISH tests with centromeric or locus-specific probes

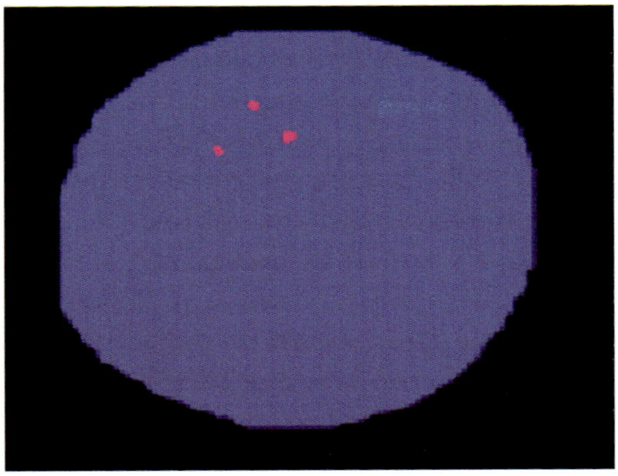

Fig. 3: FISH with Vysis DNA probe LSI 21/ spectrum orange showing three signals for trisomy 21 for chromosome 21 aneuploidy. (DNA: deoxyribonucleic acid; FISH: fluorescence in situ hybridization)

include five common aneuploidy detection for trisomies of 13, 18, and 21 and the sex chromosomes, targeted microdeletion syndromes like 22q11.2 deletion, Williams syndrome, and translocations involving various subtelomeres. Whole paint probes can help to delineate subtle suspected translocations on metaphase obtained from cultured cells. Cytogenetic evaluation of some structurally abnormal chromosomes, e.g., marker chromosomes is also possible in some cases. The sensitivity (83–100%) and specificity (99.8–100%) of interphase prenatal FISH tests has been summarized from multiple report (Shaffer et al., 2007). This should depend on the quality of the probes and preparation of samples for hybridization.

Sample

Same as for karyotype.

Indications of Fluorescent in situ Hybridization in Fetal Medicine

- As an adjunct to karyotype or microarray for a quick targeted result
- For a specific microdeletion syndrome.

Limitations

It requires prior knowledge of the specific chromosomal abnormality to be investigated. It is not a comprehensive test for all possible chromosomal abnormalities and it is usually used as an adjunct to a complete chromosomal analysis evaluation. These rapid aneuploidy detection (RAD) tests are adjunctive to the complete diagnostic tests of karyotyping or CMA.

Multiplex Ligation-dependent Probe Amplification

Multiplex ligation-dependent probe amplification is a DNA-based multiplex assay to detect deletions and duplications referred to as copy number variations (CNVs) in the chromosome or genes of the human genome.

Sample

Deoxyribonucleic acid-based test—blood in ethylenediaminetetraacetic acid (EDTA) coagulant vacutainer, fetal samples, and product of conception.

Indications

This method is used for identification of single or more than one exon deletions and duplications as in Duchenne muscular dystrophy **(Fig. 4)** and SMN1 and SMN2 copy numbers as in spinal muscular atrophy. Methylation-specific multiplex ligation-dependent probe amplification is used to determine methylation as well as copy number defects as for Angelman, Prader–Willi, Beckwith–Weidman, Silver–Russel syndromes as well as methylation of CpG islands in fragile X. A special type of MLPA called subtelomeric MLPA examines the common subtelomeric regions of all chromosomes which are known to cause recurrent deletions and duplications.

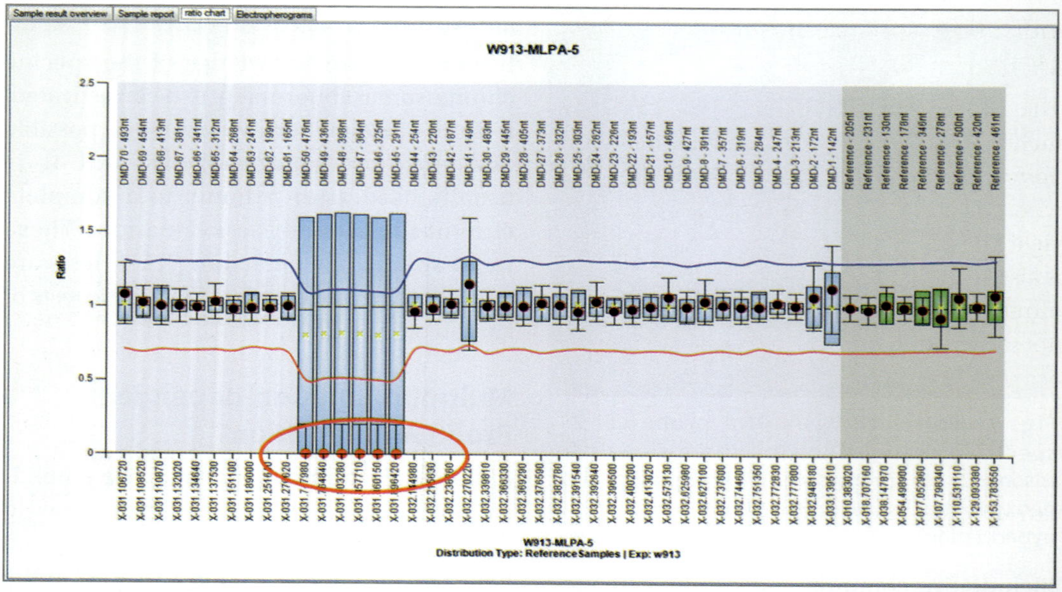

Fig. 4: Multiplex ligation-dependent probe amplification (MLPA) ratio plot showing hemizygous deletion of exon 45–50 in a male patient with Duchenne muscular dystrophy. Deletions are highlighted as red dots.

Limitations

This test will not identify balanced translocations, all unbalanced translocations, and single-variant nucleotide mutations in genes causative of disease.

Chromosomal Microarray Analysis

This technique enables the study of chromosomes at a higher resolution than gold standard karyotype. In simple terms, CMA is a multiplex FISH with hundreds and thousands of labeled oligonucleotides and SNPs from all over the genome. The number of probes used on the immobilized array slides on which the patient's DNA is hybridized with a differentially labeled dye and identifies chromosomal or genomic regions that are deleted or duplicated of at least 1,000 bp size, referred to as CNVs. This requires computerized software as the number of probes are many and cannot be assessed manually or microscopically. CMA has the ability to detect genomic deletions up to 20 kb and duplications up to 40 kb. The sensitivity and specificity of detection of the DNA dosage imbalances detected are dependent on the size of the CNV and the coverage and density of the clone of probes of the platform used for this test. Various databases (ClinVar, ClinGen, Decipher, UCSC, etc.) and published literature are used to interpret the CNVs as pathogenic, benign, and variations of uncertain significant (VUS). The benefit of CMA is that it interrogates various regions of the whole genome for pathogenic and benign CNVs at a much higher resolution than other cytogenetic and molecular cytogenetic tests.

Sample

DNA-based test—blood in EDTA coagulant vacutainer, fetal samples, and product of conception.

Indications for Chromosomal Microarray Analysis

The indications of this test in fetal medicine include evaluation of a fetus with ultrasound abnormalities or multiple malformations where it has a 6–10% additional diagnostic yield compared to a karyotype analysis. CMA is also a very good technique for stillbirth and intrauterine death as the testing method does not require dividing cells. Even in the absence of a structural malformation in the fetus, it can provide additional information in 1–2% (16–18). Another indication for CMA in the fetal sample is when a parent is a heterozygous carrier of a balanced translocation.

Limitations

The limitation of a microarray includes the VUS for which literature evidence is not available. Therefore, expert genetic counseling is mandatory to help appropriate parental decisions for the pregnancy. A CMA is not the test of choice for monogenic disorders.

Case

The first pregnancy of a nonconsanguineously married couple—the anomaly scan identified fetal growth restriction, congenital cardiac malformation, and agenesis of corpus callosum. There was a family history on the paternal side of recurrent pregnancy losses. A fetal sample was tested for chromosomal CNVs by CMA. A 5.0 Mb deletion of chromosome 6p25.3p25.1 and a 23.8 Mb duplication of chromosome 4p16.3p15.2 was identified in the fetal sample **(Figs. 5A and B)**. In view of this report, a parental karyotype analysis was advised and performed and the father was identified to have a balanced chromosomal translocation between chromosome 4 and 6. The parents were rendered genetic counseling with details of about the options for future pregnancies.

BEYOND CHROMOSOMES, DISORDERS DUE TO GENE MUTATIONS

Case

A 27-year-old second gravida has one 4-year-old child with transfusion-dependent beta thalassemia major. She provides this history in her first antenatal history at 8 weeks gestation. What will be the genetic counseling provided and flow of events for this family?

Beta thalassemia major is a disorder that occurs due to a mutation in both copies of the beta thalassemia gene, *HBB*. This is an autosomal recessive disorder that occurs due to mutations/variations in both copies of the *HBB* gene in the affected child. The parents are carriers in that one of their two copies have the mutation and thereby, they do not have any disease manifestations.

The steps for prenatal diagnosis for this family include:

- Confirming the clinical diagnosis in the proband and the carrier status in the parents
- Polymerase chain reaction-(PCR)-based testing or *HBB* gene sequencing in the proband and parents to identify the gene mutation causing the disorder in this family **(Figs. 6A to C)**.
- Genetic counseling to explain the about the disorder, recurrence risk, option of prenatal testing, procedure, risks, and limitations of the same.
- The specific mutation in the family must be identified prior to prenatal diagnostic procedure. In the fetal sample, the specific mutation relevant to the family is tested.

This *direct detection of the specific DNA variant* in the prenatal sample is the method

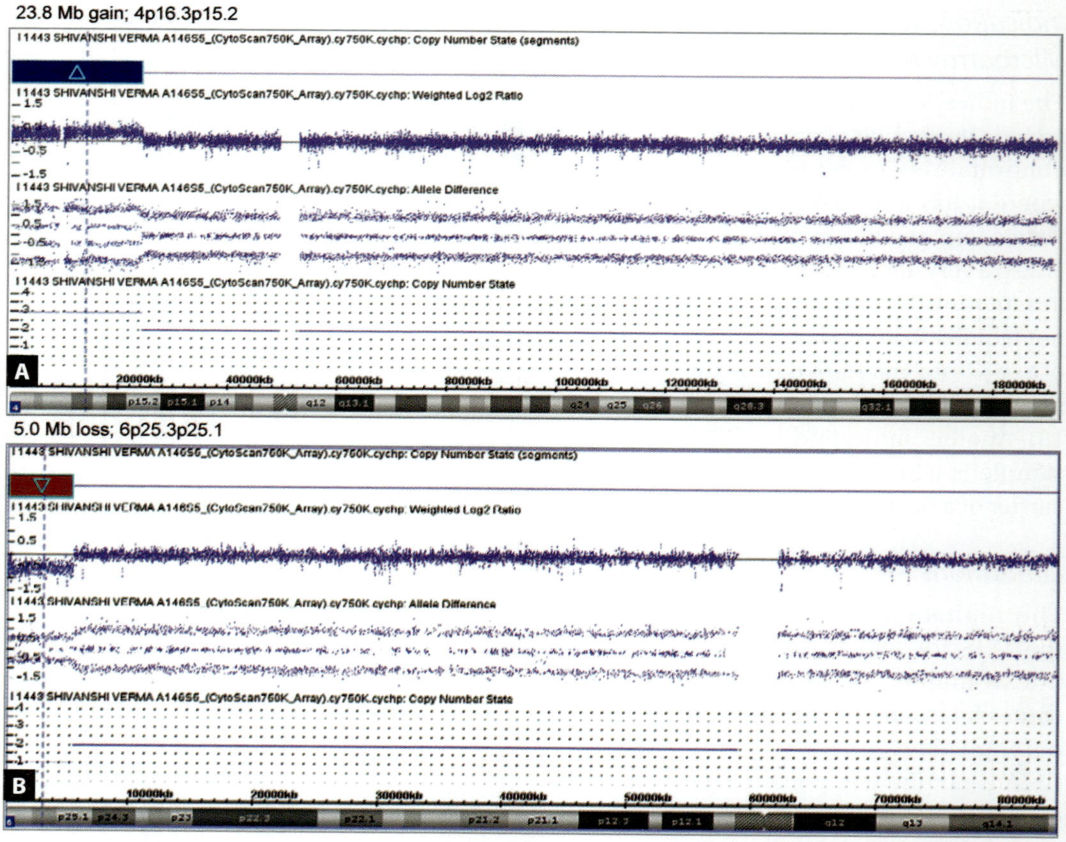

Figs. 5A and B: arr[GRCh37] 4p16.3p15.2(68346_23955546)x3, 6p25.3p25.1(381118_5402772)x1.

of choice in all cases with a previously affected child or when a targeted disease-causing DNA variant is known in the couple. A DNA variant is defined as a nucleotide change from the reference sequence. These are simple, low throughput, most accurate diagnostic PCR-based tests.

The *PCR-based methods* can be applied for many disorders including beta thalassemia, sickle cell anemia, achondroplasia, myotonic dystrophy, fragile X syndrome, Huntington disease, etc.

It is important to check for *maternal cell contamination* in the fetal sample as it can result in erroneous reporting of the fetus. Maternal cell contamination is ruled out by quantitative fluorescent PCR (QF-PCR) of various microsatellite markers present on the various chromosomes **(Figs. 7A and B)**.

TRIPLET-REPEAT DISORDERS

The expansion of a tandemly repeated trinucleotide sequence, cytosine, adenine, and guanine (CAG), is the mutational mechanism for several human genetic diseases such as myotonic dystrophy, Huntington's disease, fragile X, Friedreich ataxia, and spinocerebellar ataxias. Detection of expansion employs PCR amplification method using a fluorescently labeled locus-specific primer, flanking the CAG/CGG/GAA, etc. repeats together with paired primers

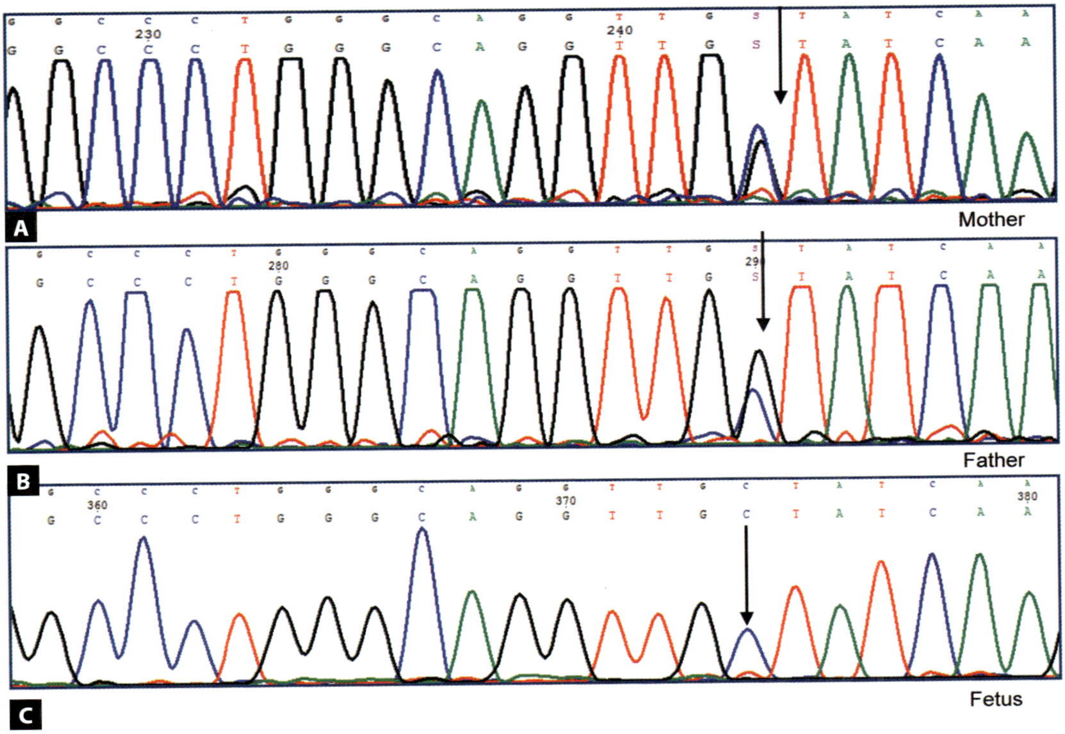

Figs. 6A to C: Partial chromatogram of *HBB* gene. Both mother and father are heterozygous for IVS 1–5 G > C (c.92 + 5 G > C) and fetus is homozygous (both alleles with the same DNA change) for IVS 1–5 G > C (c.92 + 5 G > C). Mutation is marked by arrows.

amplifying from multiple priming sites within the repeats. Triplet-repeat primed PCR (TP PCR) gives a characteristic ladder on the fluorescence trace, enabling the rapid identification of large pathogenetic repeats that cannot be amplified using flanking primers **(Fig. 8)**.

NEXT-GENERATION SEQUENCING

Next-generation sequencing is a high throughput method of analysis of a large number of genes together on one platform and at one time. This technique is very good for disorders or phenotypes that occur due to mutations in any one of many genes, e.g., Noonan disorder and RASopathies, hypertrophic cardiomyopathy, and ciliopathy group of disorders. The options available when using this technology include testing all 20,00 genes (ES), testing only those genes that are relevant to the phenotype (panel testing), or testing all genes for which there is disease phenotype correlation, about 5,000 genes of the Online Mendelian Inheritance in Man (OMIM morbid genes) as a clinical exome. The variant identified by this test is assigned a pathogenic, likely pathogenic, benign, likely benign, and variant of unknown significance category based on standard criteria for variant interpretation and classification.

Exome sequencing interrogates about 1.5–2% of the genome and includes testing for mutations in only the exons. This test

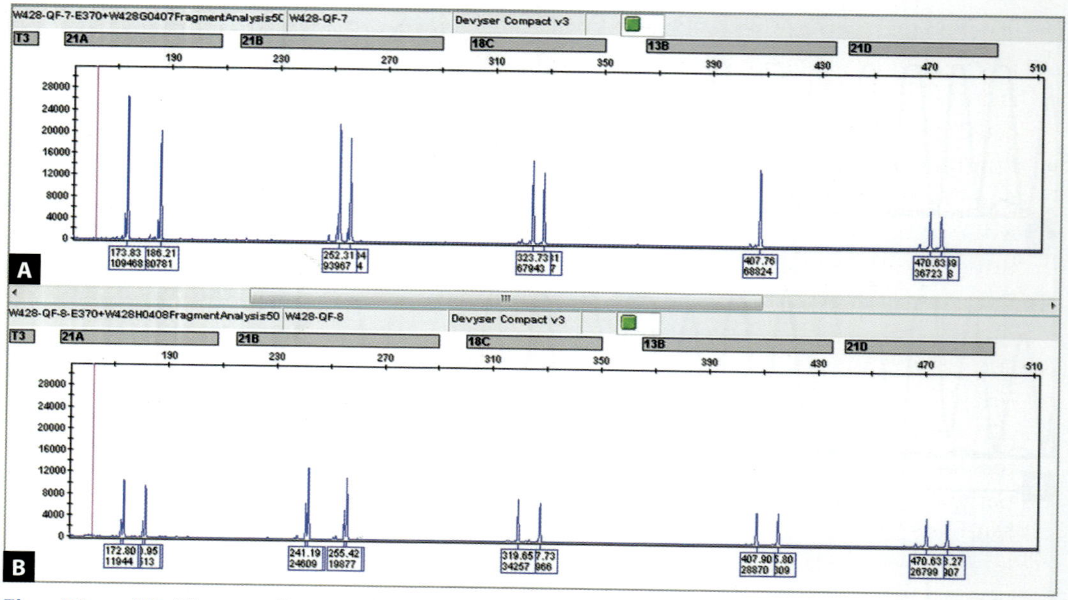

Figs. 7A and B: Microsatellites marker analysis of mother (A) and fetus (B). The presence of only one maternal allele in the fetal sample indicates the absence of MCC and confirms that the sample is a pure fetal DNA sample and the accuracy of PND is reliable. (DNA: deoxyribonucleic acid; MCC: maternal cell contamination; PND: prenatal diagnosis)

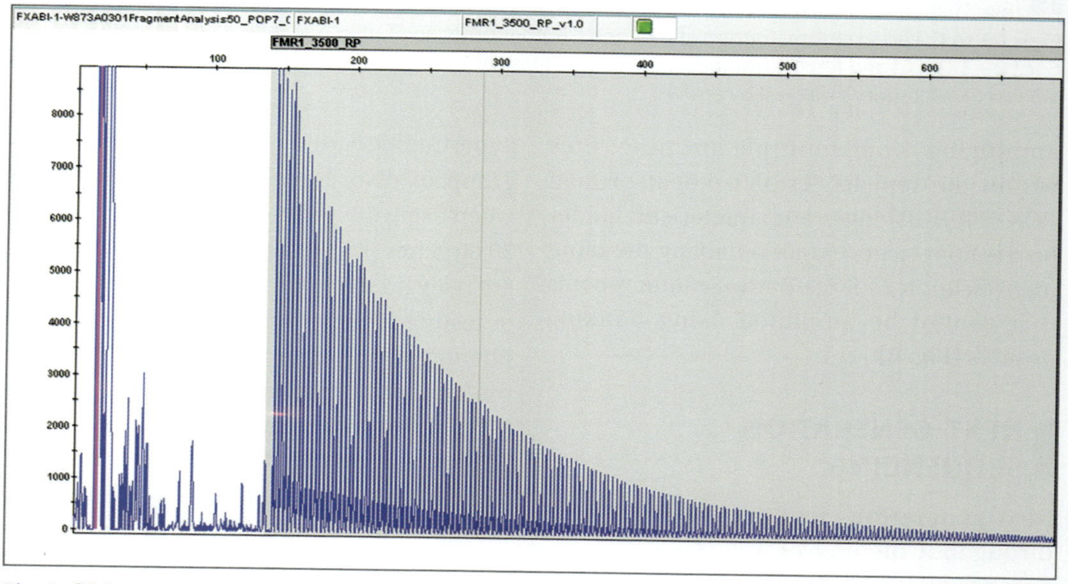

Fig. 8: CGG repeat expansion detected by triplet-primed polymerase chain reaction (PCR) in a male sample.

is indicated for use in the presence of fetal anomalies with normal CMA. Some salient features of this are highlighted further.

- Trio prenatal ES (pES) of fetus and parents is preferred to allow for timely pathogenic variant evaluation. If solo pES is performed, segregation of the identified pathogenic/likely pathogenic variants is important before assigning them as causative of fetal phenotype.

- Limited information of fetal genotype–phenotype correlation
- Adequate and detailed clinical information is to be provided to the laboratory while ordering the test. This includes detailed fetal imaging reports such as sonograms, magnetic resonance imaging (MRI), and/or fetal cardiac ultrasound, prior fetal prenatal test results, and/or clinical laboratory report, parental past medical history, ethnicity, reproductive history, and family history, including parental consanguinity.
- Pretest and post-test genetic counseling is best provided by trained personnel or geneticists who understand the phenotype and can apply the appropriate test for the clinical situation, interpret the test results and explain to the family as per guidelines. Informed consent is to be undertaken before genetic testing for any fetal indication.
- Turnaround time—needs to be rapid during pregnancy and is best.
- The greatest challenge of pES is the variants of unknown significance identified on sequencing. Great experience and expertise is required to analyze these variants.
- The laboratory performing the genomic tests must be accredited and have experience in variant interpretation and fetal phenotype correlation.

At the present time, there are no data supporting the clinical use for ES for other reproductive indications, such as the identification of sonographic markers suggestive of aneuploidy or a history of recurrent unexplained pregnancy loss.

Indications of Prenatal Exome Sequencing in Fetal Medicine

- Multiple fetal malformations with normal CMA or single major malformation suggestive of a genetic disorder
- Fetal malformations highly specific of a single gene disorder, e.g., rhabdomyoma
- Family history of a monogenic disorder
- Severe fetal growth restriction with normal CMA
- Increased nuchal translucency with normal CMA.

Limitations of Prenatal Exome Sequencing

- Variants of uncertain significance (VOUS) are difficult to interpret due to evolving fetal phenotype.
- There is always a race against time due to turnaround time being more than 3 weeks.
- There is possibility of a blending of two or more phenotypes, wherein pES evaluation is very challenging.

As these genomic technologies are rapidly developing, these statements need to be reviewed frequently.

Case

Consanguineous family with second-affected child with short long bones and decreased bone density suggestive of osteogenesis imperfecta (OI) on the level II scan. OI is a skeletal dysplasia caused by mutations in more than one gene. This is referred to as genetic heterogeneity. Recurrence in a consanguineous family is most likely due to an autosomal recessive inheritance. A close differential diagnosis for OI is hypophosphatasia, a similar autosomal recessive disorder. Postnatal treatment is available for both disorders with variable outcomes. The couples are counseled and the above details discussed with them. In this clinical scenario, the option of pES can be offered to confirm the diagnosis and genotype-phenotype correlation of informed counseling **(Figs. 9 and 10)**.

A pictorial representation of the confirmatory prenatal tests with indications of each is summarized in **Figure 10**. A summary of the prenatal tests with advantages and disadvantages of each is summarized in **Table 1**.

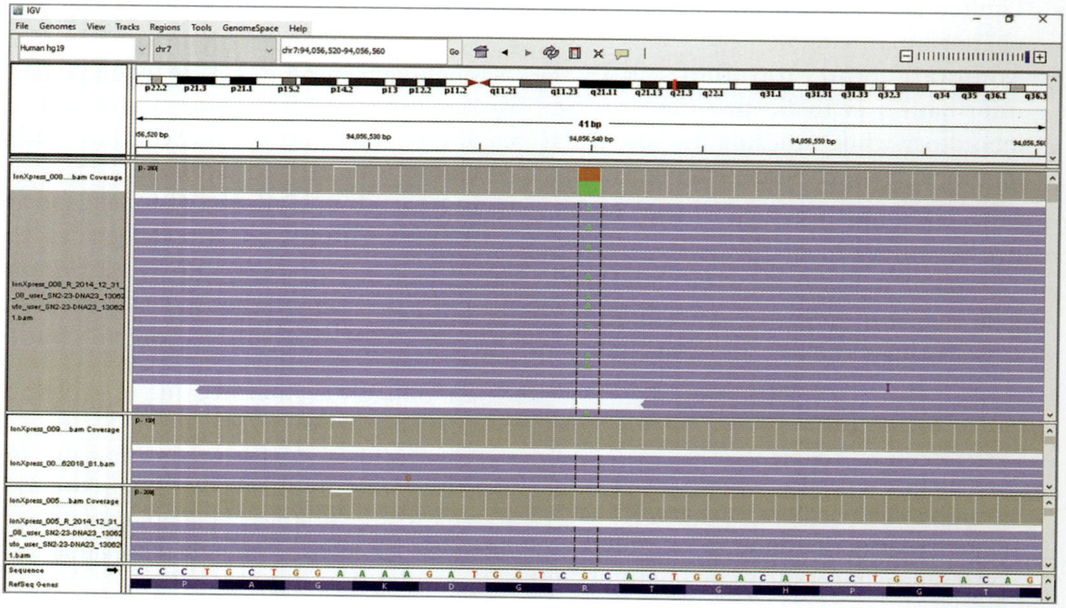

Fig. 9: Integrative Genomics Viewer (IGV) snapshot showing heterozygous variant: c.3200G > A; p.(Arg1067His) in *COL1A2* gene.

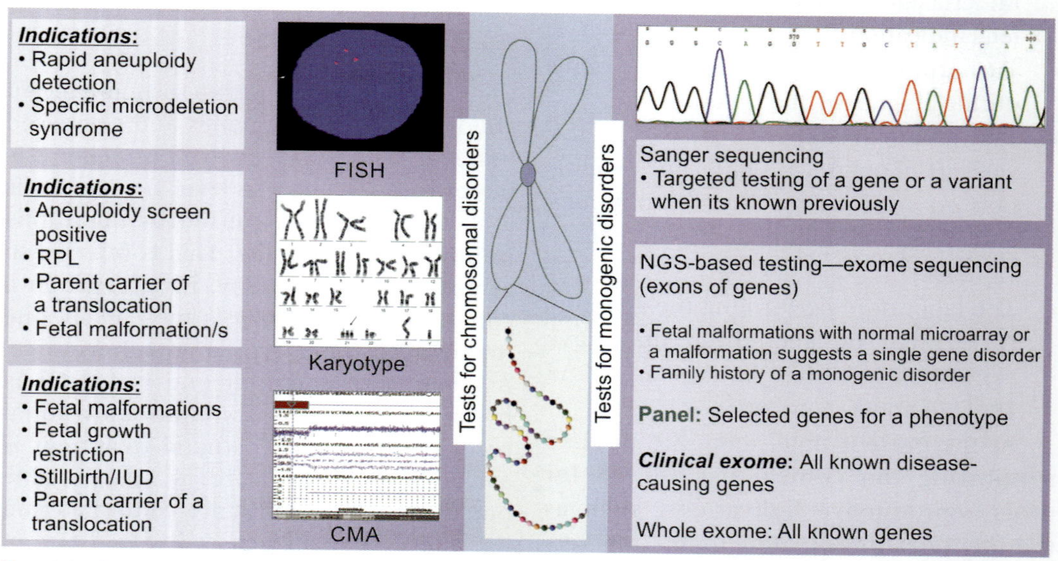

Fig. 10: Genetic tests in prental diagnosis at glance. (CMA: chromosomal microarray analysis; FISH: fluorescence in situ hybridization; IUD: intrauterine death; NGS: next-generation sequencing; RPL: recurrent pregnancy loss)

TABLE 1: Different testing methodologies, indications, advantages, and limitations.

Test name	Detection spectrum	Reporting time	Resolution	Advantages	Limitations	Indications in prenatal testing
Karyotype	*Chromosomal abnormalities*: Loss/gain of chromosomal material, inversions, translocations, ring chromosomes, isochromosome, marker, mosaicism	2–3 weeks	>5–10 Mb	• Gold standard test for aneuploidies, polyploidies, and other structural aberrations • Affordable	Cannot detect microdeletions, microduplications, and very low-level mosaicism, or maternal cell contamination	• Risk for trisomy 21, 13, and 18 on antenatal screening tests • Advanced maternal age • Fetal malformations consistent with a specific chromosomal disorder • Family history of a chromosomal disorder • Positive cffDNA screen
FISH	Targeted areas of the genome	2–3 days	0.5 Mb	Quick results	Expensive, needs targeted probes, cannot screen all genomic regions together, does not detect maternal cell contamination	• Rapid aneuploidy testing • Specific microdeletion disorder, e.g., 22q11.2 microdeletion syndrome, can be used for validation of CNVs found in CMA
CMA	Chromosomal abnormalities	7–10 days	20 kb losses 40 kb gains	Detects small deletions or duplications, characterizes abnormalities such as markers and ring	Cannot detect balanced translocation or cannot differentiate between free trisomy 21 or translocation Down syndrome. Some platforms miss triploidy	• Fetal malformations • Multiple soft markers • Family history of chromosomal disorders • As an adjuvant to FISH or QF-PCR, it gives an additional 2% of diagnostic yield when performed for patients with normal USG

Contd...

Contd...

Test name	Detection spectrum	Reporting time	Resolution	Advantages	Limitations	Indications in prenatal testing
MLPA	Exon/gene deletions and duplications	5 days	Exon level	Gold standard for exon level CNVs. Can detect methylation	• Commercial kits not available for all genes • Not detect balanced rearrangements or SNVs	• Family history of DMD, SMA, Alpha thalassemia • Subtelomeric MLPA for RPL
Direct DNA variant detection	SNVs, triplet-repeat disorders	1–2 weeks	Base pair level	Cheap, gold standard for the specific pathogenic variant	Requires a prior pathogenic variant identified in the family	Family history of a genetic disorder or one/both partners are carriers of a pathogenic genetic variant
Sanger sequencing	SNVs	1–2 weeks	Base pair level	Gold standard for SNV detection	Suitable for small genes. Does not identify deletions/duplications	Beta thalassemia, connexin 26 related deafness, achondroplasia, hypochondroplasia
Exome	Monogenic disorders	3–6 weeks	Base pair level	Picks up SNVs, small deletions and duplications in coding region	Does not identify large CNVs, triplet-repeat disorders, methylation disorders, balanced rearrangements	• Multiple fetal malformations with normal CMA • Fetal malformations highly specific of a single-gene disorder • Severe FGR with normal CMA

(cffDNA: cell-free fetal deoxyribonucleic acid; CMA: chromosomal microarray analysis; CNVs: copy number variations; DMD: Duchenne muscular dystrophy; FGR: fetal growth restriction; FISH: fluorescent in situ hybridization; MLPA: multiplex ligation-dependent probe amplification; QF-PCR: quantitative fluorescent polymerase chain reaction; RPL: recurrent pregnancy loss; SMA: spinal muscular atrophy; SNVs: single nucleotide variants; USG: ultrasonogram)

SUGGESTED READING

1. ACOG Technology Assessment in Obstetrics and Gynecology No. 14. Modern Genetics in Obstetrics and Gynecology. Obstet Gynecol. 2018;132(3):e143-68.
2. American College of Obstetricians and Gynecologists' Committee on Practice Bulletins—Obstetrics; Committee on Genetics; Society for Maternal-Fetal Medicine. Screening for Fetal Chromosomal Abnormalities: ACOG Practice Bulletin, Number 226. Obstet Gynecol. 2020;136(4):e48-69.
3. Dugoff L, Norton ME, Kuller JA; Society for Maternal-Fetal Medicine (SMFM). The use of chromosomal microarray for prenatal diagnosis. Am J Obstet Gynecol. 2016;215(4):B2-9.
4. Hui L, Ellis K, Mayen D, Pertile MD, Reimers R, Sun L, et al. Position statement from the International Society for Prenatal Diagnosis on the use of non-invasive prenatal testing for the detection of fetal chromosomal conditions in singleton pregnancies. Prenat Diagn. 2023;43(7):814-28.
5. Jenkins M, Seasely AR, Subramaniam A. Prenatal genetic testing 1: screening tests. Curr Opin Pediatr. 2022;34(6):544-52.
6. Jenkins M, Seasely AR, Subramaniam A. Prenatal genetic testing 2: diagnostic tests. Curr Opin Pediatr. 2022;34(6):553-8.
7. Phadke SR, Puri RD, Ranganath P. Prenatal screening for genetic disorders: Suggested guidelines for the Indian Scenario. Indian J Med Res. 2017;146(6):689-99.
8. Practice Bulletin No. 162: Prenatal Diagnostic Testing for Genetic Disorders. Obstet Gynecol. 2016;127(5):e108-22.
9. Stevens B. Impact of Emerging Technologies in Prenatal Genetic Counseling. Cold Spring Harb Perspect Med. 2020;10(12):a036517.

9

CHAPTER

Approach to Common Fetal Abnormalities

Chanchal Singh, Harshiba Kaur

KEY POINTS

1. Incidence of congenital abnormalities is 2–3% in general population.
2. Ultrasound remains the primary imaging modality for detecting structural anomalies. The introduction of the first-trimester anomaly scan has allowed much earlier detection of these anomalies.
3. First- and second-trimester screening offer valuable information on chromosomal and genetic abnormalities. Most common congenital defects are cardiac defects (8–10/1,000 live birth) followed by neural tube defects [(4–11.4/1,000 live births (LBs)].
4. Counseling should be nondirective and accurate regarding the likely clinical condition, association with genetic disorders and outcomes including long term outcomes and maternal risks in case an intervention is planned.
5. Invasive prenatal diagnostic techniques are reserved for cases requiring definitive diagnosis. Amniocentesis or chorionic villus biopsy can be done as per the gestational age and fetal deoxyribonucleic acid (DNA) can be analyzed by karyotyping, microarray or whole exome sequencing.
6. Multidisciplinary collaboration is vital in managing fetal abnormalities and ensuring the best possible outcomes in cases amenable to therapy such as meningomyelocele.
7. Fetal therapy and intervention may be considered in select cases to improve the prognosis such as fetal shunts in cases of lower urinary tract obstruction (LUTO) and fetoscopic endoluminal tracheal occlusion (FETO) in cases of congenital diaphragmatic hernia (CDH).
8. Ethical considerations and parental support are critical aspects of managing pregnancies with fetal abnormalities.
9. There is also continuous research ongoing in the field of fetal therapy, and some modalities, like in utero repair of severe open neural tube defects, can now be offered wherever facilities are available.

INTRODUCTION

Fetal structural abnormalities may be seen in 2–3% of all pregnancies. Although there is a lack of surveillance of congenital defects in our country, published literature reports a higher prevalence. It is estimated that 1.7 million birth defects occur annually, with congenital heart defects being the most common abnormalities (8–10/1,000 LBs) followed by neural tube defects (4–11.4/1,000 LBs).[1] Congenital abnormalities remain a leading cause of stillbirth and neonatal deaths and constitute a huge burden, especially in low-middle-income countries like ours where potential treatment and rehabilitation are not accessible and affordable to all.[2] Thus, prenatal screening and diagnosis play an important role in counseling parents, pregnancy decision-making, and planning delivery at the appropriate center where facilities for postnatal care and treatment are available. This chapter aims to provide an overview of the common fetal anomalies and a clinical approach to their management.

ETIOLOGY

Structural abnormalities may be associated with exposure to teratogens, e.g., anti-epileptic drugs, or may result from exposure to infections like rubella. They may also be associated with chromosomal abnormalities or monogenic disorders with variable modes of inheritance or can be multifactorial resulting from a combination of environmental and genetic factors.

PRENATAL DIAGNOSIS

Ultrasound remains the mainstay for antenatal detection of structural abnormalities. The detection rates vary according to the organ system involved; e.g., the prenatal detection for open neural tube defects is nearly 100%, whereas abnormalities like an imperforate anus and isolated ear anomalies have very poor antenatal detection. The detection rates are also influenced by the operator experience, the quality of the ultrasound machine, and patient-specific factors like the maternal body mass index (BMI), multiple pregnancy, oligohydramnios, etc. The best detection rates are achieved, however, functional defects cannot be known on USG by performing the ultrasound according to a prespecified protocol. These protocols are laid down by international bodies like the International Society of Ultrasound in Obstetrics and Gynecology (ISUOG) and Fetal Medicine Foundation (FMF). Every hospital should have its own predefined anomaly screening protocol. A good USG can reduce but not eliminate the chance of birth defects.

Mid-trimester Anomaly Scan

Mid-trimester anomaly scan is the main ultrasound for the detection of structural abnormalities. It is performed at 18–22 weeks of gestation, preferably between 20 and 22 weeks and with good equipment and in expert hands majority of clinically important structural abnormalities can be detected at this time. However, detection rates vary widely between centers and operators. The highest detection rates are achieved when ultrasound is performed by trained operators according to a prespecified protocol. The proposed images that should be obtained at this scan are given in **Figures 1A to P**. Detection rates also vary according to the type of anomaly; e.g., detection rates for open neural tube defects are >90%, whereas detection rates for cardiac defects are <50%. Even in western countries with an established screening protocol, detection rates in low-risk populations are about 50%.

First-trimester Screening

First-trimester screening has traditionally been synonymous with screening for Down syndrome. However, it has now increasingly been recognized as an opportunity for early detection of many structural abnormalities. The first-trimester scan has moved beyond just viability, dating, confirming the number of fetuses, and aneuploidy screening to detecting anomalies in the very beginning. The new guidelines recommended by ISUOG 2023 require the complete fetal structure to be evaluated.[3] **Figures 2A to L** illustrate the images required to be taken in the first-trimester scan.

Approximately 50% of the structural anomalies can be diagnosed in the first

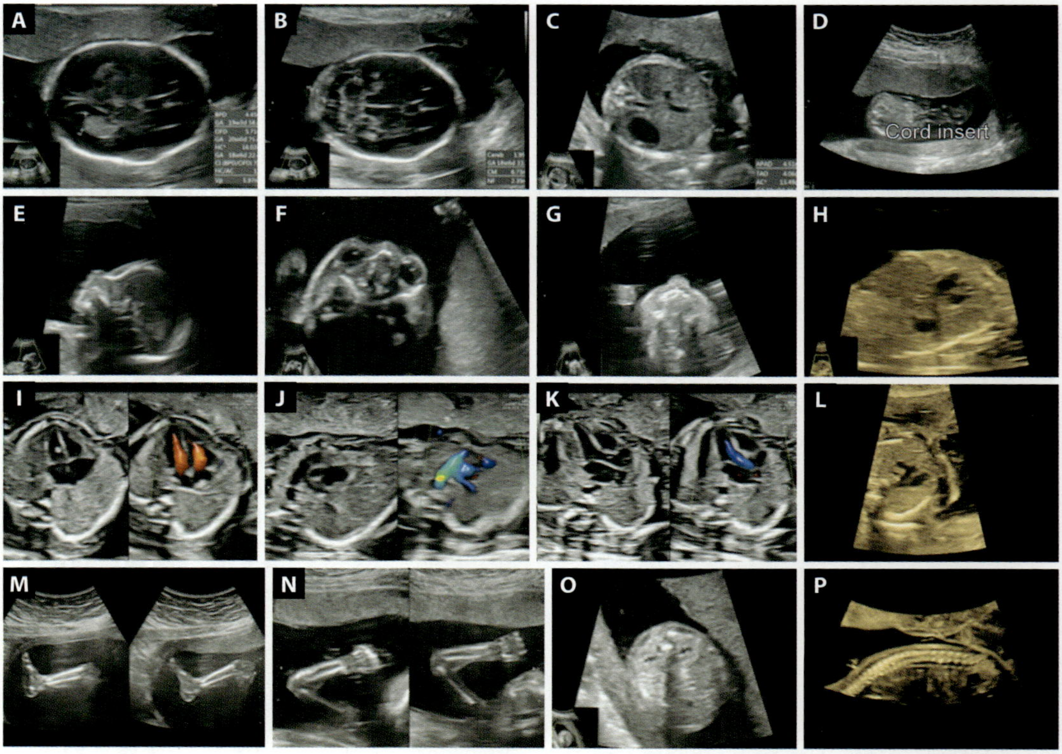

Figs. 1A to P: Proposed images to be obtained at a second-trimester anomaly scan.

trimester itself.[4-6] The advantages of this approach are that, firstly, lethal anomalies like acrania-anencephaly and holoprosencephaly can be offered termination in the first trimester, which can reduce maternal risks, and secondly, enough time is at hand for prenatal testing and diagnosis when certain anomalies that require further workup are detected.[7] However, the first-trimester anomaly scan does not replace a detailed second-trimester targeted scan for fetal anomalies. Many anomalies suspected in the first trimester may need a confirmation for definitive diagnosis in the second trimester. **Figures 3 and 4** provide examples of potentially detectable abnormalities in the first trimester.

A routine anomaly scan is done at 18–20 weeks.[8] **Figures 1A to P** show the proposed planes to be taken in all mid-trimester anomaly scans.

ABNORMALITIES THAT MAY PRESENT IN THE THIRD TRIMESTER

About 1.6% of structural abnormalities may present in the third trimester (with a previously normal mid-trimester anomaly scan), e.g., bowel abnormalities, CDH, trachea-esophageal fistulas, coarctation of aorta, certain brain abnormalities, and intracranial hemorrhage, and parents should be counseled regarding these. All couples must also be counseled that all structural abnormalities cannot be detected prenatally. Some factors like maternal habitus, multiple pregnancy, oligohydramnios may limit

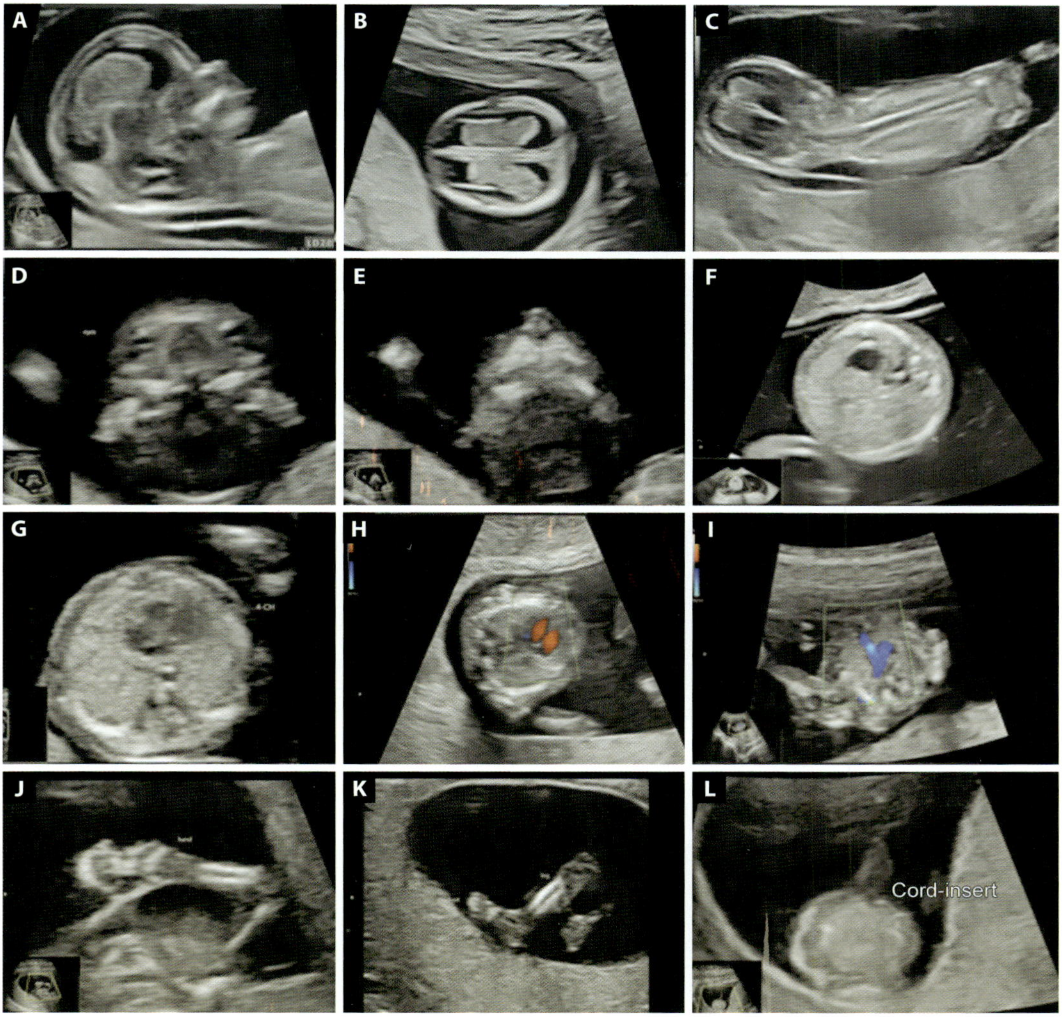

Figs. 2A to L: Images that should be obtained at the first-trimester ultrasound.

the detection rates. Fetal position must be documented while reporting.

DIAGNOSTIC WORKUP

A thorough personal and family history may reveal the presence of structural anomalies in the family. These must always be elicited by drawing a three-degree pedigree chart. A complete physical examination should be done for both parents as it may reveal stigmata of some dominantly inherited conditions, e.g., tuberous sclerosis, central incisor, features suggestive of 22q deletion syndrome, etc. Once an abnormality is diagnosed on ultrasound, the patient should be referred to a fetal medicine center for confirmation of diagnosis and a detailed ultrasound, including fetal echocardiogram, to rule out other associated abnormalities should be done. Invasive diagnostic testing

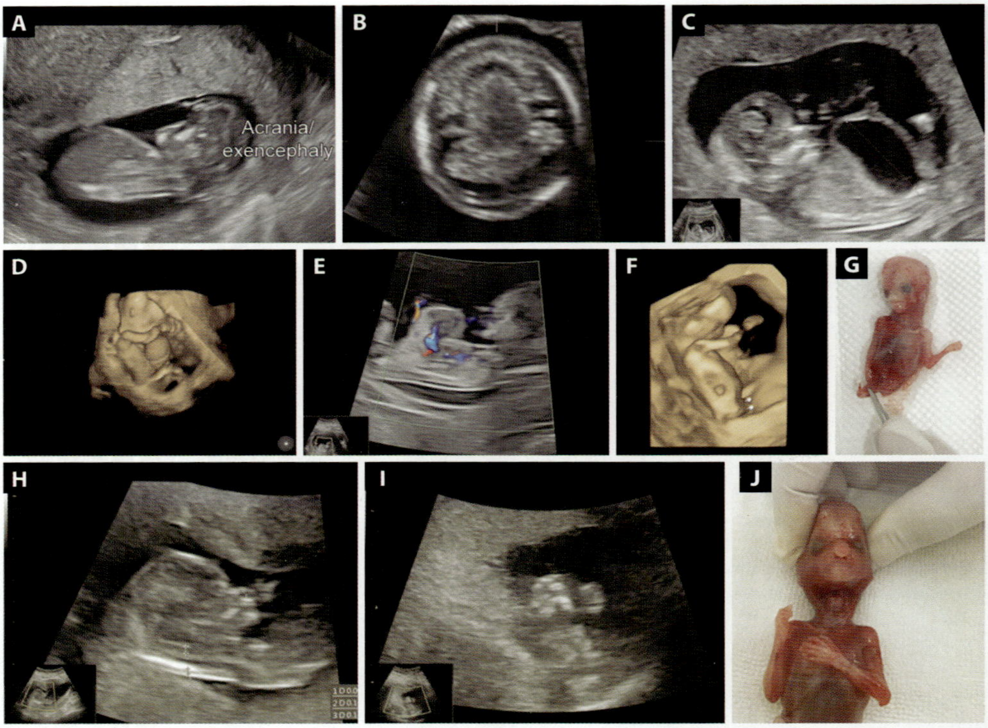

Figs. 3A to J: Potentially detectable abnormalities in first trimester. (A) Acrania/exencephaly; (B) Holoprosencephaly; (C) Megacystis; (D and E) Exomphalos; (F and G) Caudal regression syndrome; (H, I, and J) Bilateral cleft lip and palate.

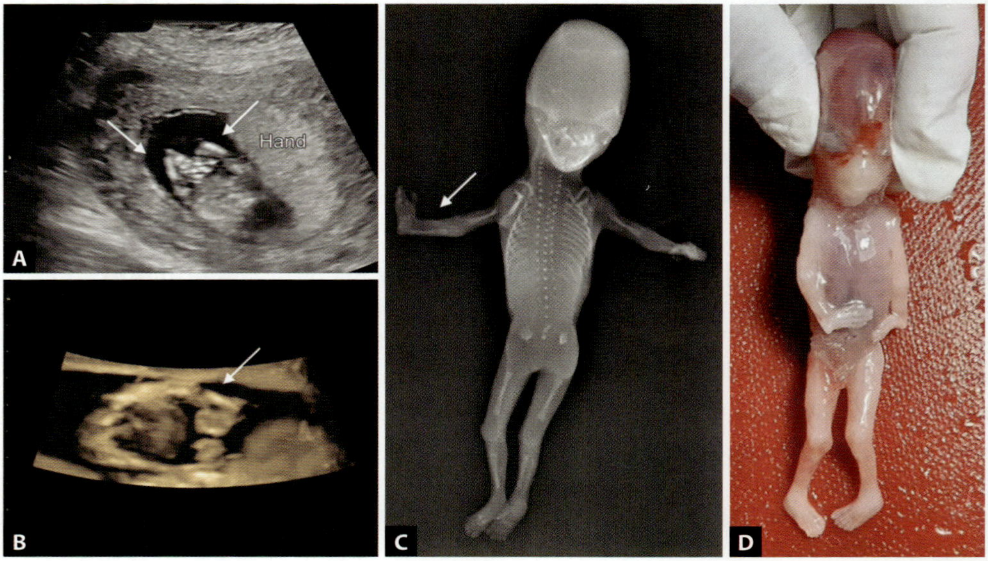

Figs. 4A to D: Bilateral radial aplasia detected in the first trimester.

TABLE 1: Workup on detection of a fetal structural abnormality.

	Parental	*Fetal*
History	• Consanguinity • Fever with rash • Radiation exposure • Medications, e.g., warfarin, antiepileptic drugs, ACE inhibitors, etc. • Alcohol intake • Substance abuse • Family history of genetic disorders • Three-generation pedigree	
Examination	Autosomal dominant traits relevant to specific conditions, e.g., central incisor, features suggestive of 22q deletion, etc.	• Detailed anomaly scan • Fetal echo • MRI if indicated • Review ultrasound after 3–4 weeks to look for evolving features
Investigations	• Maternal TORCH IgM, IgG • Maternal blood sugar, HbA1c • *Parental genetic testing as indicated:* – Karyotype – Microarray – Exome	*Invasive diagnostic testing:* • Chorionic villus sampling • Amniocentesis • Fetal blood sampling

[ACE: angiotensin converting enzyme; HbA1c: glycated hemoglobin; Ig: immunoglobulin; MRI: magnetic resonance imaging; TORCH: toxoplasmosis, others (syphilis, hepatitis B), rubella, cytomegalovirus, herpes simplex]

should be offered to the patient as many structural abnormalities may be associated with chromosomal abnormalities. The couple should be counseled that the risk of miscarriage associated with these procedures in experienced hands is as low as 0.5%. It is currently recommended that microarray should be offered in place of conventional karyotype because of the 6% incremental increase in the yield of pathogenic copy number variants (CNVs) over the common aneuploidies. A follow-up scan after 3–4 weeks should be scheduled as there may be evolving features or abnormalities that may manifest at a later gestation. Fetal magnetic resonance imaging (MRI) can be used as an adjunct for better imaging in case of high maternal BMI, oligohydramnios, or for better imaging of fetal brain, lung, gastrointestinal disorders, etc. **Table 1** summarizes the workup required on detection of a fetal abnormality.

MANAGEMENT

If the abnormality is correctable postnatally and the parents opt for expectant management, they should be managed in a multidisciplinary unit with joint counseling by a maternal-fetal medicine (MFM) specialist, geneticist, neonatologist, and the relevant subspecialty, e.g., pediatric cardiology, pediatric surgery, pediatric nephrology, etc. Serial ultrasounds and follow-up antenatal visits should be arranged. Delivery should be planned in a tertiary care center with neonatal intensive care unit (NICU) and pediatric subspeciality services. Delivery should be aimed at term with the mode of delivery to be individualized according to the obstetric and fetal factors.

If the abnormality is lethal and/or the parents opt for termination of pregnancy, it is essential to counsel them regarding fetal autopsy before termination for a detailed phenotyping which involves both external and internal examinations. They should be counseled regarding genetic testing and DNA storage postnatally. These are essential to confirm the diagnosis, identify a possible etiology, and assign recurrence risk in subsequent pregnancies. Autopsy should be performed by a trained perinatal pathologist or medical geneticist.

The approach to a pregnancy when diagnosed with a structural abnormality is summarized in **Flowchart 1**.

Some fetal abnormalities may be amenable to prenatal therapy, e.g., fetal thoraco-amniotic shunt for pleural effusion associated with fetal solid lung lesions like congenital pulmonary airway malformation (CPAM), in utero fetal meningomyelocele repair, fetal tracheal occlusion in cases of congenital diaphragmatic hernia, FETO in cases of congenital diaphragmatic hernia, and fetal vesicoamniotic shunt for LUTO. These may not be available in the country, e.g., FETO, or at all centers. The couple should be given nondirective accurate counseling regarding the procedure and its outcomes, including long-term outcomes and maternal risks (in both current pregnancy and future pregnancies) following the procedure. Local complication rates should be used in

Flowchart 1: Approach to pregnancy with fetal structural abnormality, fetal therapy, and intervention.

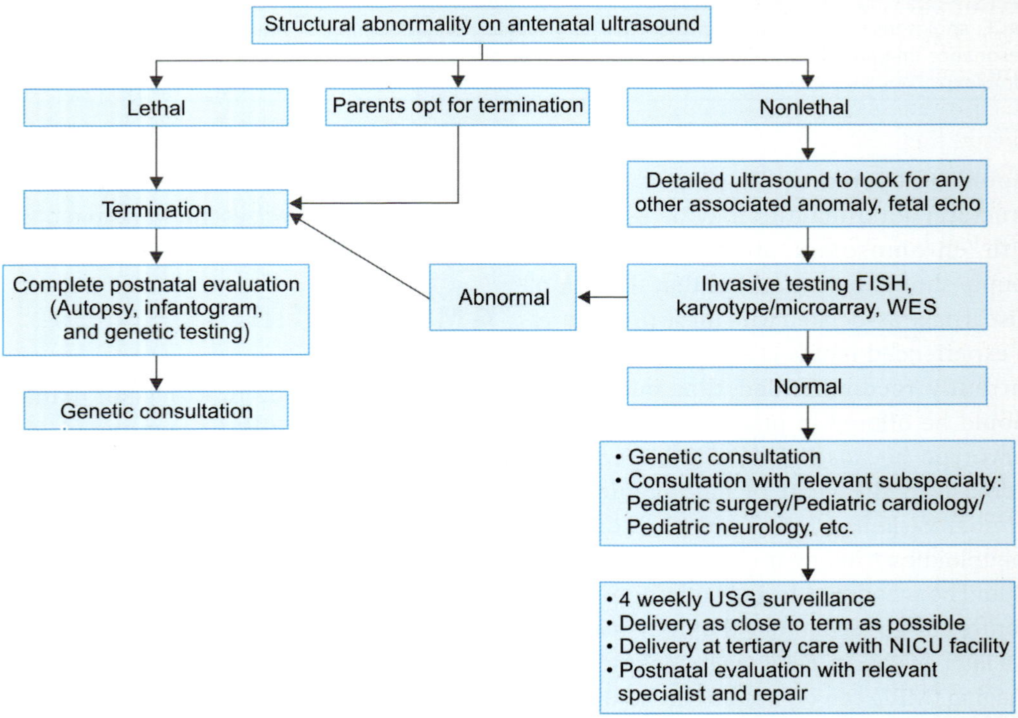

(FISH: fluorescence in situ hybridization; NICU: neonatal intensive care unit; USG: ultrasonography; WES: whole exome sequencing)

counseling wherever the procedure is being planned.

FETAL PROGNOSIS AND LONG-TERM OUTCOMES

Anomalies like anencephaly, severe hydrocephalous, hypoplastic left heart syndrome, and bilateral renal agenesis are lethal, and pregnancy termination should be offered in these cases. Some nonlethal anomalies may progress in severity which may worsen the fetal prognosis in late gestation, e.g., congenital diaphragmatic hernia or large cystic lung malformations. These fetuses need to be monitored at regular intervals and counseled appropriately.

ETHICAL CONSIDERATIONS

The recent amendment of the Medical Termination of Pregnancy (MTP) Act in 2021 has extended the gestational age limit for termination of pregnancy. This has provided relief to women who have missed their early antenatal care and lethal fetal anomalies or anomalies that have the potential to severely affect the mental and physical health of the child and have been detected late. These women can be offered termination of pregnancy till 24 weeks of gestation. The termination must be approved by two practicing gynecologists between 20 and 24 weeks. There is a clause in the new amendment, which also allows termination of such severe anomalies beyond 24 weeks, after approval of the Institute Medical Board, which constitutes a group of experts including but not limited to an obstetrician, neonatologist, radiologist, and geneticist.

PREVENTION

Although most of the isolated structural abnormalities are sporadic and the risk of recurrence remains low, the presence of multiple ultrasound findings/anomalies might indicate a syndrome that may be inheritable. When such inheritable conditions are found in the pedigree, genetic consultation is a must. Appropriate tests like microarray and whole exome sequencing can be offered to the index case along with the couple, which may provide a basis for prenatal diagnostic testing in the subsequent pregnancy. Universal supplementation with folic acid in the dose of 400 μg should be offered to all women planning conception. This has been found to be effective in reducing the risk of neural tube defects. Women with a history of a previous child with neural tube defects should be given a higher dose of folic acid (4 mg/day).

REFERENCES

1. Bhide P, Gund P, Kar A. Prevalence of congenital anomalies in an Indian maternal cohort: Healthcare, prevention, and surveillance implications. PLoS One. 2016;11(11):e0166408.
2. Bhide P, Kar A. A national estimate of the birth prevalence of congenital anomalies in India: systematic review and meta-analysis. BMC Pediatr. 2018;18(1):175.
3. International Society of Ultrasound in Obstetrics and Gynecology; Bilardo CM, Chaoui R, Hyett JA, Kagan KO, Karim JN, Papageorghiou AT, et al. ISUOG Practice Guidelines (updated): performance of 11-14-week ultrasound scan. Ultrasound Obstet Gynecol. 2023;61(1):127-43.
4. Singh C, Shahnaz G, Dagar S, Shastri A, Kurana D, Thakur S. Performance of first-trimester ultrasound in detection of structural abnormalities in Indian women: A prospective observational study. Int J Gynaecol Obstet. 2023;160(3):1042-3.
5. Karim JN, Roberts NW, Salomon LJ, and Papageorghiou AT. Systematic review of first-trimester ultrasound screening for detection

of fetal structural anomalies and factors that affect screening performance. Ultrasound Obstet Gynecol. 2017;50(4):429-41.

6. Goley SM, Sakula-Barry S, Adofo-Ansong N, Isaaya Ntawunga L, Tekyiwa Botchway M, Kelly AH, et al. Investigating the use of ultrasonography for the antenatal diagnosis of structural congenital anomalies in low-income and middle-income countries: a systematic review. BMJ Paediatr Open. 2020; 4(1):e000684.
7. Syngelaki A, Chelemen T, Dagklis T, Allan L, Nicolaides KH: Challenges in the diagnosis of fetal non-chromosomal abnormalities at 11- 13 weeks. Prenat Diagn. 2011;31:90-102.
8. Salomon LJ, Alfirevic Z, Berghella V, Bilardo CM, Chalouhi GE, Da Silva Costa F, et al. ISUOG Practice Guidelines (updated): performance of the routine mid-trimester fetal ultrasound scan. Ultrasound Obstet Gynecol. 2022;59(6):840-56.

10 CHAPTER

Abdominal Malformations

Manisha Kumar

KEY POINTS

Fetal abdominal malformations are generally detected late in gestation. There is possibility of evolution of the anomaly; hence, follow-up ultrasound evaluation is needed.

1. *Omphalocele:* Diagnostic feature is umbilical cord insertion into the membrane covering the abdominal wall defect. The risk of chromosomal abnormality is high up to 40%; hence, chromosomal testing should be advised. Outcome is good if isolated and liver is not completely herniated.
2. *Gastroschisis:* Diagnostic feature is presence of bowel loops freely floating in the amniotic fluid. Risk of chromosomal abnormalities is very low.
3. *Duodenal atresia:* Sonographic diagnosis is made by appearance of "double bubble" and presence of late polyhydramnios. Risk of chromosomal abnormality is up to 30%, mainly trisomy 21. Outcome is good if isolated.
4. *Body stalk anomaly:* Diagnostic feature is the demonstration of abdominal organs in the extraembryonic celom and a short umbilical cord. Risk of chromosomal abnormalities is low, but it is uniformly fatal.
5. *Meconium peritonitis:* May be associated with infection and cystic fibrosis which is an autosomal recessive disease.
6. *Abdominal cyst:* The size and position of cyst in relation to other abdominal structures are important for prognosis.

INTRODUCTION

The intra-abdominal abnormality poses a challenge because it involves different systems and organs from gastrointestinal (GI) tract to urinary or genital structures. Generally, the abdominal malformations are detected late in gestation. Some abnormalities such as gastric or bladder emptying show variation even during the course of same ultrasound (US) examination.

ABDOMINAL WALL DEFECTS

Anterior abdominal wall defects are roughly classified into three types: Gastroschisis, omphalocele, and body stalk-like anomalies. Body stalk anomaly is the rarest, most severe and invariably lethal abdominal wall defect.

Omphalocele (Box 1)

- Omphalocele is a defect in the abdominal wall closure involving cord insertion.
- It is among the more common anterior abdominal wall defects; studies have estimated that the overall prevalence ranges from 2 to 3 per 10,000 births worldwide.[1]
- The defect is thought to be caused by an abnormality that occurs during the process of body infolding at 10–12 weeks of gestation.[2]

Ultrasound Findings and Diagnosis

- The ultrasonographic appearance of omphalocele varies depending on the size and location of the defect; however, a principal diagnostic feature of omphalocele is the umbilical cord insertion into the membrane covering the abdominal wall defect **(Fig. 1)**.

- The cord insertion site at the caudal apical portion of the omphalocele membrane can be visualized with color flow Doppler studies on sagittal or oblique images. An additional diagnostic feature is the presence of the intrahepatic portion of the umbilical vein coursing through the central portion of the defect **(Fig. 1)**.
- Occasionally, the membrane covering of the omphalocele might rupture. In these cases, the abdominal contents lie floating free in the amniotic cavity, similar to gastroschisis. However, unlike gastroschisis, in ruptured omphalocele, the defects are usually large and have exposed liver.
- *Omphaloceles may be stratified into three groups:* Small, giant, and ruptured. A giant omphalocele (GO) is one with an abdominal wall defect size >5 cm or with >50% or 75% of the liver within the sac.[3] Although GO has surgically poor prognosis, they are less often associated with chromosomal abnormality.
- Omphalocele is associated with elevated maternal serum alpha-fetoprotein (MSAFP) levels.

BOX 1: Omphalocele.

- *Diagnostic feature:* Umbilical cord insertion into the membrane covering the abdominal wall defect
- *Risk of chromosomal abnormalities:* High up to 40%
- *Risk of nonchromosomal syndromes:* High OEIS (omphalocele, bladder exstrophy, imperforate anus, and spina bifida) complex, Beckwith–Wiedmann syndrome
- *Outcome:* Good if isolated and liver is not completely herniated, poor if liver is found herniated in the sac **(Fig. 2)**

Prognosis and Management

- Once identified, a sonographic estimation of the size of the omphalocele, contents of the omphalocele sac, location of the umbilical cord insertion relative to the herniation, and the presence of an aminoperitoneal membrane should be documented.
- Up to 70% of omphalocele cases are associated with other structural malformations, chromosomal abnormalities, and genetic syndromes and this phenomenon is significantly associated with the ultimate prognosis for these

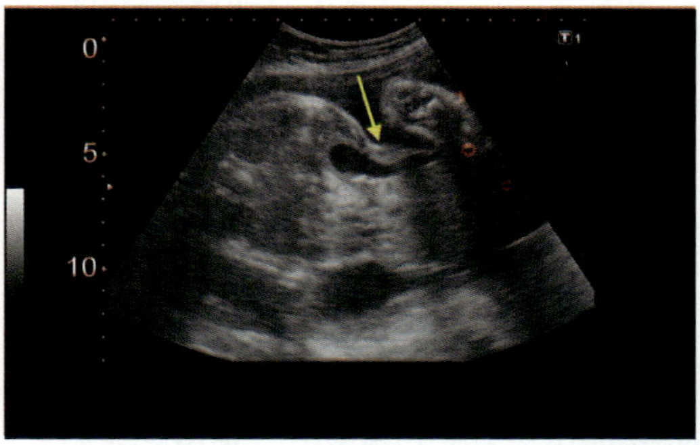

Fig. 1: Protrusion from anterior abdominal wall with covering membrane and cord over it in the axial section of fetal abdomen on ultrasound (US).

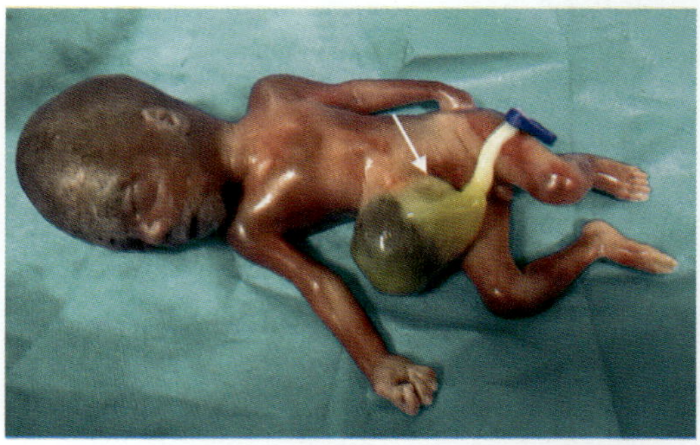

Fig. 2: The baby with omphalocele with liver in the contents; cord can be seen attached at the top.

fetuses.[4] A careful sonographic search for other fetal anomalies should also be performed, including fetal echocardiography. Chromosomal analysis is strongly recommended.

- Comprehensive counseling should be done by the specialists in pediatric surgery, genetics, neonatology, and pediatric cardiology.

Postnatal Management

- The survival rate of isolated omphalocele is as high as 96%.[5] The goal of the management of fetuses with omphalocele is to deliver the fetus as close to term as possible. Delivery should occur in a tertiary care center with neonatologists available for immediate resuscitation.
- Initial treatment consists of airway stabilization and sterile wrapping of the abdominal defect to preserve heat and minimize insensible fluid loss. A complete physical examination should be performed to rule out a syndromic diagnosis.
- Management of the omphalocele consisted of primary closure of the defect depending on its size and peak inspiratory pressures during the surgical procedure. If at all possible, primary fascial closure is the preferred method of repair because of a lower incidence of sepsis, biliary obstruction, and fistula and a reduced number of operations and rate of mortality in patients who undergo this repair.[6]
- For very large omphaloceles, a staged reduction using a prosthetic silo is preferred.

Gastroschisis (Box 2)

Gastroschisis (Greek for belly cleft) is a full-thickness defect in the abdominal wall that occurs secondary to incomplete closure of the lateral folds during the 6th week of gestation. It may occur as a result of a malformation, disruption, or deformation.[8]

BOX 2: Gastroschisis.

- *Diagnostic feature:* Bowel loops freely floating in the amniotic fluid
- *Risk of chromosomal abnormalities:* Very low
- *Risk of nonchromosomal syndromes:* Low Gastrointestinal anomalies may be associated in 20–40% of cases[7]
- *Outcome:* Very good

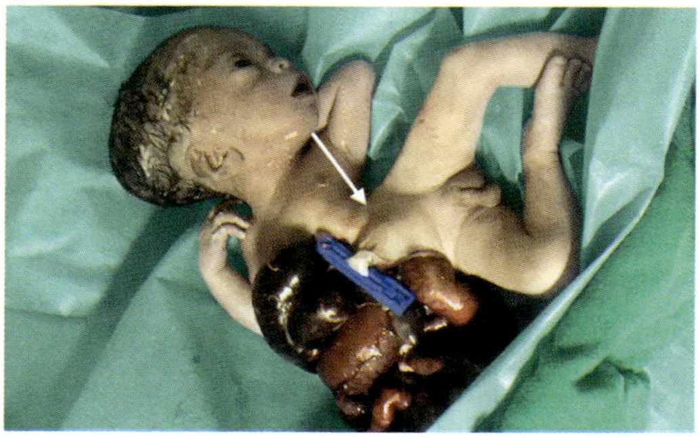

Fig. 3: Abdominal wall defect in the baby was seen on the right of cord insertion; there was no membrane covering and the cord is inserted at its normal position.

Ultrasound and Diagnosis

- In gastroschisis, the US shows the abdominal wall defect immediately to the right of the normal umbilical cord insertion into the abdominal wall **(Fig. 3)**.
- In contrast to omphalocele, gastroschisis is usually not associated with extra GI abnormalities or chromosomal abnormality. This may be the reason for the better outcome of gastroschisis.
- However, GI anomalies may be associated in 20–40% of cases. These include malrotation, atresia, volvulus, and infarction.[9]

Prognosis and Management

- Fetuses with gastroschisis are at risk for a number of complications that directly affect survival during the newborn period. Obstetric complications include intrauterine growth restriction, which can affect up to 77% of fetuses.[10]

- Other obstetric complications include preterm labor which occurs in over one third of cases due to associated polyhydramnios. Abnormalities of amniotic fluid volume, both polyhydramnios and oligohydramnios, can accompany gastroschisis.[9]

Postnatal Management

- The condition of the bowel at the time of birth is the single most important factor affecting long-term outcome of fetuses with gastroschisis. The extent of bowel damage is variable in gastroschisis and can range from only mild to severe, with bowel atresia and necrosis requiring resection with staged repair. Most of the damage is caused by constriction at the site of the abdominal wall defect and that this occurs primarily late in gestation.
- At birth, the eviscerated bowel characteristically has a thick edematous appearance described by a "peel."[8] The peel involves the serosa and is composed of fibrin and collagen. The peel in gastroschisis is thought to be caused by exposure to amniotic fluid combined with constriction at the abdominal wall defect.[8] In baby with gastroschisis, conservative managed is provided till stabilization **(Fig. 4)**.
- Gastroschisis has been generally considered a sporadic event, with a multifactorial cause.

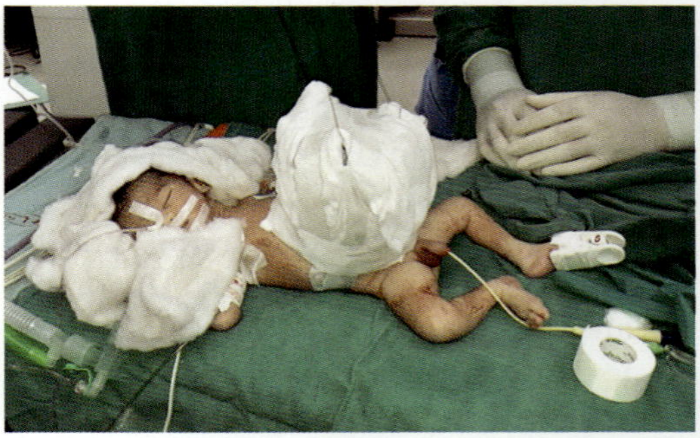

Fig. 4: Live baby with gastroschisis being managed conservatively till stabilization.

Body Stalk Anomaly (Box 3)

- Body stalk anomaly is a severe abdominal wall defect that results from abnormalities in the development of the cephalic, caudal, and lateral embryonic body folds.

BOX 3: Body stalk anomaly.

- *Diagnostic feature:* Demonstration of abdominal organs in the extraembryonic celom and a short umbilical cord
- *Risk of chromosomal abnormalities:* Low
- *Risk of nonchromosomal syndromes:* Variety of conditions may be associated, including the amniotic band syndrome, short umbilical cord syndrome, and limb–body wall complex
- *Outcome:* Uniformly fatal

- This maldevelopment results in the absence or shortening of the umbilical cord with the abdominal organs lying outside the abdominal cavity and directly attached to the placenta.[11]
- The variety of phenotypes in the reported cases worldwide has led to the creation of a confusing array of terms for this condition including the amniotic band syndrome, short umbilical cord syndrome, and limb–body wall complex.

Ultrasound and Diagnosis

- The criteria for the diagnosis of body stalk anomaly in the first trimester includes demonstration of abdominal organs in the extraembryonic celom and a short umbilical cord with only two vessels.[12]
- The diagnosis may be more difficult to make during the second trimester than

during the first because of the presence of severe oligohydramnios.

- If the diagnosis of body stalk anomaly is certain, chromosomal analysis is not indicated, as all reported cases have been associated with a normal karyotype.
- The differential diagnosis for body stalk anomaly includes isolated omphalocele, isolated gastroschisis, short umbilical cord syndrome, and limb-body wall complex.
- Some authors consider body stalk anomaly to be a severe form of amniotic band syndrome. Amniotic bands are present in 40% of cases of body stalk anomaly.[13]
- In addition, some of the limb defects that can be associated with body stalk anomaly can be attributed to amniotic bands. Limb-body wall complex is included in the spectrum of defects seen in the early amnion rupture sequence **(Figs. 5A and B)**.[12]

Prognosis and Management

- If the diagnosis of body stalk anomaly is made, termination of pregnancy should be offered as the condition is uniformly fatal in a newborn.
- Abnormal fetal presentation is common; therefore, there are increased chances of cesarean section.

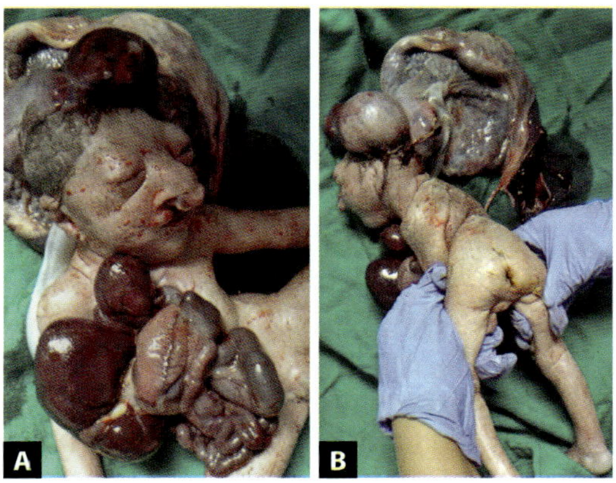

Figs. 5A and B: Abdominal wall defect and a very short cord with encephalocele and facial cleft; the cord is extremely short and placenta is seen attached to the head.

DUODENAL ATRESIA (BOX 4)

- In duodenal atresia, the tract between proximal and distal portions of duodenum is atretic; it is one of the most common prenatally diagnosed GI anomalies.
- It may be due to interruption of vascular supply during organogenesis or may be because of failure of recanalization of the solid stage during early embryogenesis.
- Duodenal stenosis or atresia occurs in approximately 1 in 10,000 live births.[7]

Ultrasound and Diagnosis

- Duodenal atresia is suspected when there is presence of polyhydramnios, which is present in more than half of the cases.[14] Prenatal sonography may show the characteristic "double bubble" sign that represents the dilated fluid-filled stomach and proximal duodenum **(Figs. 6A and B)**.[15]
- The double bubble sign usually appears late in the gestation and duodenal atresia may present as dilated stomach early in gestation.

BOX 4: Duodenal atresia.

- *Incidence:* 1 in 6,000 live births.
- *Diagnosis:* Sonographic diagnosis is made by appearance of "double bubble" and presence of late polyhydramnios
- *Risk of chromosomal anomalies:* High 30%, mainly trisomy 21
- *Risk of other anomalies:* As there is high risk of heart abnormality, fetal echocardiography is also advised
- *Outcome:* Good if isolated

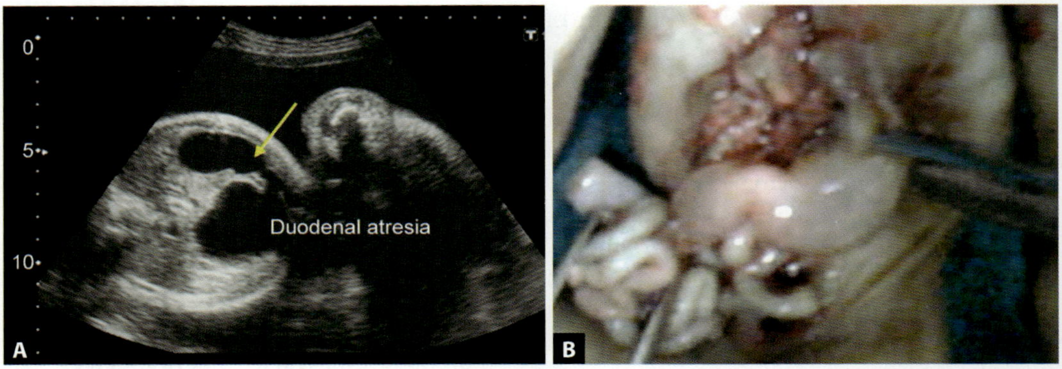

Figs. 6A and B: Axial view of abdomen on ultrasound (US) on the left, showing double bubble, with a communication between the stomach and dilated proximal duodenum. The autopsy picture on the right showing constriction at the distal part of duodenum, shown by the arrow.

- Care should be taken to demonstrate the communication between the two bubbles to demonstrate that the second bubble is the proximal dilated part of duodenum.
- As 30% of patients with duodenal atresia will have trisomy 21, other sonographic features of Down syndrome should be sought, including nuchal fold thickening, hypomineralization of fifth-finger middle phalanx (clinodactyly).[16]
- Atresia is more common than stenosis and occurs in approximately 70% of cases.[15]
- Skandalakis et al. have described three types of duodenal atresia. The most common duodenal anomaly (69% of cases) is membranous mucosal atresia (type I) with an intact muscular wall. The proximal duodenum is ballooned out, while the duodenum distal to the atresia is narrowed.[15]
- A type II duodenal atresia is rare (2% of cases) and has a short fibrous cord connecting the two ends of the atretic duodenum.
- Type III duodenal atresia has a complete separation between the two ends of the duodenum and can be associated with biliary tract anomalies in 6% of cases also.
- Duodenal stenosis accounts for the remaining 23% of cases. These anatomic relations are rarely evident sonographically.[15]
- Annular pancreas occurs in 20–30% of patients with duodenal atresia or stenosis.[17] Annular pancreas can produce extrinsic compression and result in stenosis, but it is more commonly associated with an intrinsic obstruction due to complete atresia.

Antenatal Management and Prognosis

- If duodenal atresia is suspected, the fetus should undergo genetic amniocentesis because of the high incidence of associated chromosomal anomalies.
- Fetal echocardiography should also be performed to evaluate possible associated congenital heart anomalies, even in the presence of a normal karyotype. Early detection of associated anomalies may influence decisions regarding continuation of the pregnancy.
- Polyhydramnios can contribute to the development of preterm labor.

- Pediatric surgical consultation with parents should be offered to help alleviate anxiety and to provide answers to questions concerning postnatal intervention.
- Delivery should be planned in a center with appropriate neonatal and pediatric surgical support.

Postnatal Management

- The surgical reconstruction is usually performed on the day of delivery after the infant is assessed for the presence or absence of associated anomalies and appropriate volume resuscitation and correction of electrolyte disturbances.
- The surgery performed is either excision of an intrinsic web or more commonly duodeno-duodenostomy or a duodeno-jejunostomy.

ABDOMINAL CYST (BOX 5)

Most antenatally diagnosed fetal abdominal cysts are ovarian in origin. Though most disappear antenatally, nearly three quarters required surgical intervention when present after birth. Cysts of intestinal origin are more difficult to diagnose antenatally and often require surgery.

BOX 5: Distinctive characteristics of abdominal cyst.

- Ovarian cysts are located at one side of the bladder, round in shape, and are observed in female fetuses
- Choledochal cysts are located in the hilar, are oblong or oval in shape, and are connected to the bile duct
- Intestinal duplication cyst is located in the middle of abdomen, close to the intestine, and present as an intestinal wall-like structure
- Mesenteric cysts are round in shape with thin tensionless wall, present as multiple chambers and are easily deformable on compression

Ultrasound and Diagnosis

- Regardless of the underlying pathology, the most common sonographic presentation is that of a round, anechoic structure of variable size and position **(Fig. 7)**.
- One of the main difficulties after identifying a cyst is establishing its origin.
- Excluding urinary origin, the most common etiologies of fetal intra-abdominal cysts are: Ovarian cysts, GI cystic duplication, hepatic and biliary tree cysts, meconium pseudocysts, mesenteric cysts, adrenal cysts, splenic cysts, and hydrometrocolpos.[18]
- The differential diagnosis can be aided by knowledge of the sex of the fetus, the location, the appearance, and the relationship with the adjacent structures of the cyst, as well as the prevalence of the various etiologies.[18]

Antenatal Management and Prognosis

- The most challenging problem is to decide which cases will be amenable to US monitoring, postnatal surgery, or even prenatal invasive therapy.

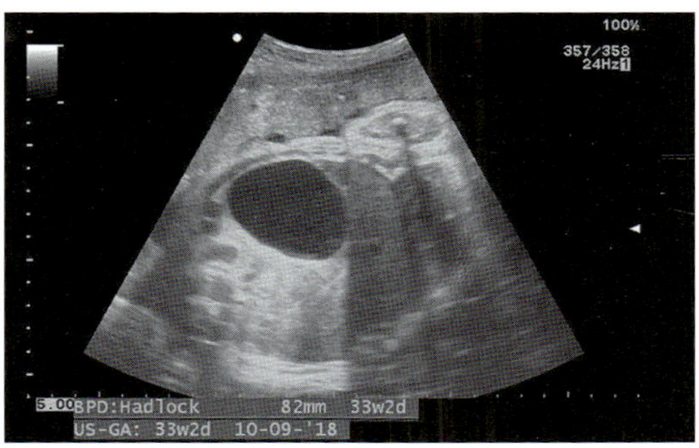

Fig. 7: Ultrasound (US) shows a large anechoic cystic structure, above the bladder to one side of fetal abdomen.

- Fetuses with intra-abdominal cystic lesion should be followed sonographically for the development of polyhydramnios, in the majority of cases as consequence of GI malformation, and the subsequent increased risk of associated preterm labor.
- The rate of prenatal spontaneous resolution of fetal intra-abdominal cysts has been reported between 19 and 34.7%.[18]
- Fetal intra-abdominal cysts rarely require prenatal aspiration with the exception of ovarian cysts.
- Decision-making is usually based on the conclusions of multidisciplinary meetings and on the opinion of pediatric surgeon regarding postnatal management.

Postnatal Management

- Postnatal surgical intervention rate ranges from 18 to 29%.[18]
- Neonatal outcome of fetal intra-abdominal cysts is generally favorable with a mortality rate lower than 17% in previous studies.

MECONIUM PERITONITIS (BOX 6)

- Meconium peritonitis is the most common cause of fetal intra-abdominal calcifications. It is a sterile chemical peritonitis that occurs due to antenatal perforation of the bowel.

BOX 6: Meconium peritonitis.

- *Incidence:* 1 in 35,000 live births
- *Diagnosis:* Peritoneal calcifications as continuous line in the border of peritoneum, with scattered calcification throughout the peritoneum
- *Risk of chromosomal anomalies:* Low
- *Risk of other anomalies:* Associated with cystic fibrosis
- *Outcome:* Good if simple meconium peritonitis, guarded in complex peritonitis

- Meconium peritonitis occurs in approximately 1 in every 30,000 live births.[19]
- The presence of associated anomalies is unusual and depends on the underlying cause of meconium peritonitis.
- Cystic fibrosis is reported to be the cause in only 8% of cases.[20]

Ultrasound Findings

- A spectrum of findings may be observed on prenatal sonographic examination. The most consistent finding is abdominal calcifications, which are present in 85% of cases.[21]
- The sonographic criteria used for the diagnosis of meconium peritonitis include intra-abdominal calcifications that cause acoustic shadowing not caused by solid organ, intraluminal, intravascular, biliary, or tumor calcifications.
- The clinical manifestations of meconium peritonitis depend on its underlying cause, timing, and whether or not the perforation heals spontaneously.
- The peritonitis can be localized or diffused and can lead to a fibrotic reaction with intraperitoneal calcifications.
- Other findings include polyhydramnios, fetal ascites, and bowel dilatation **(Fig. 8)**. Intra-abdominal calcifications

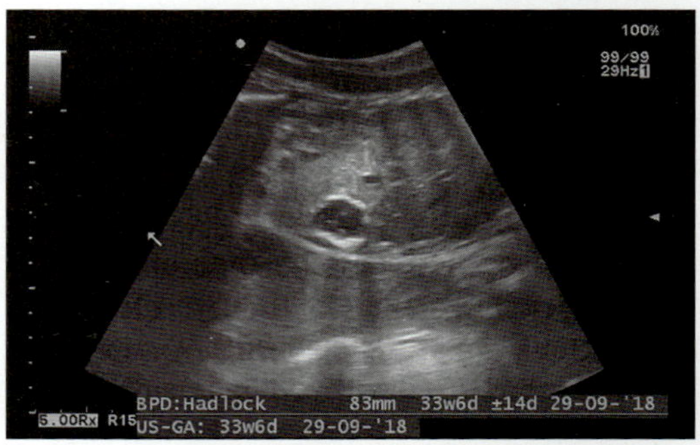

Fig. 8: Ultrasound (US) showing an irregular fetal cyst with echogenic margins with associated echogenic bowel but no ascites.

in association with any of above features are classified as complex meconium peritonitis.[22]

- Meconium peritonitis has been associated with intestinal atresia or stenosis, meconium ileus, internal hernia, bowel ileus, intussusception, gastroschisis, Meckel diverticulum, and cytomegalovirus infection.

Antenatal Management and Prognosis

- Sonographic detection of meconium peritonitis can alert the obstetrician to a fetus potentially at risk for complications from obstruction, perforation, pseudocyst formation, ascites, and polyhydramnios that may precipitate preterm labor and premature delivery.
- In the absence of the findings that characterize complex meconium peritonitis, an excellent prognosis can be anticipated.
- According to the grading system proposed by Zangheri et al., grade 0 fetuses require no surgical intervention after birth, whereas approximately 50% of grade 1 fetuses will require surgical treatment and almost all grades 2 and 3 fetuses will require postnatal surgery.[21]
- Prenatally diagnosed meconium peritonitis differs from postnatally diagnosed meconium peritonitis in reduced morbidity, lower incidence of cystic fibrosis, and an overall better prognosis. The overall mortality rate in antenatal reports is 11–14%.[22]
- Pediatric surgical consultation may be helpful in providing counseling about the overall favorable prognosis in cases of prenatally diagnosed meconium peritonitis.
- In cases of complex meconium peritonitis, the parents can be advised of a more guarded prognosis, with a 50% chance of surgical intervention during the neonatal period.[22]
- Some studies have shown that pseudocyst, intestinal loop dilatation, and ascites are predictors of the need for neonatal surgical treatment.[22] Early diagnosis and early treatment are of particular importance in neonates with fetal meconium peritonitis (FMP) complicated by intestinal perforation and obstruction.

Postnatal Management

- The infant should undergo abdominal examination immediately after delivery and an abdominal radiograph and US study of the abdomen should be obtained to confirm the prenatal findings.
- An upper GI study with small-bowel follow-through using water-soluble contrast may be necessary to confirm or exclude perforation, stenosis, atresia, or meconium pseudocysts.
- Postnatal treatment is directed by the underlying cause of meconium peritonitis.

REFERENCES

1. Gamba P, Midrio P. Abdominal Wall Defects: Prenatal Diagnosis, Newborn Management, and Long-Term Outcomes. Semin Pediatr Surg. 2014;23:283-90.
2. Sadler TW. The embryologic origin of ventral body wall defects. Semin Pediatr Surg. 2010;19:209-14.
3. Biard JM, Wilson RD, Johnson MP, Hedrick HL, Schwarz U, Flake AW, et al. Prenatally diagnosed giant omphaloceles: short- and long-term outcomes. Prenat Diagn. 2004;24: 434.
4. Fratelli N, Papageorghiou AT, Bhide A, Sharma A, Okoye B, Thilaganathan B. Outcome of antenatally diagnosed abdominal

wall defects. Ultrasound Obstet Gynecol. 2007;30:266-70.

5. Bence CM, Wagner AJ. Abdominal wall defects. Transl Pediatr. 2021;10(5):1461-9.
6. Wilson RD, Johnson MP. Congenital abdominal wall defects: an update. Fetal Diagn Ther. 2004;19(5):385-98.
7. Kucińska-Chahwan A, Posiewka A, Bijok J, Jakiel G, Roszkowski T. Clinical Significance of the Prenatal Double Bubble Sign—Single Institution Experience. Prenat Diagn. 2015; 35:1093-6.
8. Fleet MS, de la Hunt MN. Intestinal atresia with gastroschisis: A selective approach to management. J Pediatr Surg. 2000;35:1323-5.
9. Molik KA, Gingalewski CA, West KW, Rescorla FJ, Scherer LR, Engum SA, et al. Gastroschisis: a plea for risk categorization. J Pediatr Surg. 2001;36:51-5.
10. Payne NR, Simonton SC, Olsen S, Arnesen MA, Pfleghaar KM. Growth restriction in gastroschisis: quantification of its severity and exploration of a placental cause. BMC Pediatr. 2011;11:90.
11. Murphy A, Platt LD. First-trimester diagnosis of body stalk anomaly using 2- and 3-dimensional sonography. J Ultrasound Med. 2011;30:1739-43.
12. Paul C, Zosmer N, Jurkovic D, Nicolaides K. A case of body stalk anomaly at 10 weeks of gestation. Ultrasound Obstet Gynecol. 2001; 17:157-9.
13. Hunter AG, Seaver LH, Stevenson RE. Limb-body wall defect. Is there a defensible hypothesis and can it explain all the associated anomalies? Am J Med Genet A. 2011;155A:2045-59.
14. Bittencourt DG, Barini R, Marba S, Sbragia L. Congenital Duodenal Obstruction: Does Prenatal Diagnosis Improve the Outcome? Pediatr Surg Int. 2004;20:582-5.
15. Kim JY, You JY, Chang KH, Choi SJ, Oh SY, Seo JM, et al. Association Between Prenatal Sonographic Findings of Duodenal Obstruction and Adverse Outcomes. J Ultrasound Med. 2016;35:1931-8.
16. Mirza B, Sheikh A. Multiple associated anomalies in patients of duodenal atresia: a case series. J Neonat Surg. 2012;1:23.
17. Gharpure V. Duodenal atresia. J Neonatal Surg. 2014;3(1):14.
18. Sanna E, Loukogeorgakis S, Prior T, Derwig I, Paramasivam G, Choudhry M, et al. Fetal abdominal cysts: antenatal course and postnatal outcomes. J Perinat Med. 2019; 47(4):418-21.
19. Saleh N, Geipel A, Gembruch U, Heep A, Heydweiller A, Bartmann P, et al. Prenatal diagnosis and postnatal management of meconium peritonitis. J Perinat Med. 2009; 37(5):535-8.
20. Casaccia G, Trucchi A, Nahom A, Aite L, Lucidi V, Giorlandino C, et al. The impact of cystic fibrosis on neonatal intestinal obstruction: the need for prenatal/neonatal screening. Pediatr Surg Int. 2003;19(1):75-8.
21. Zangheri G, Andreani M, Ciriello E, Urban G, Incerti M, Vergani P. Fetal intra-abdominal calcifications from meconium peritonitis: sonographic predictors of postnatal surgery. Prenatal Diagnosis. 2007;27(10):960-3.
22. Shinar S, Agrawal S, Ryu M, Zani A, Chiu P, Chitayat D. Fetal meconium peritonitis—prenatal findings and postnatal outcome: a case series, systematic review, and meta-analysis. Ultraschall Med. 2020;43(2):194-203.

CHAPTER 11

TORCH Infections in Pregnancy

Suchandana Dasgupta, Poonam Tara, Shreya Singh Kushwaha

KEY POINTS

1. The nonspecific clinical presentation as well as less availability of standardized laboratories pose a challenge to correct diagnosis of TORCH infections.
2. Transmission from the mother to the fetus can occur prenatally, perinatally or postnatally.
3. The risk of affection of the fetus is greater if the infection occurs earlier in the gestational age.
4. Indications for testing include clinical symptoms in the mother, contact history, abnormal ultrasound findings of the fetus or placenta.
5. The tests include pathogen specific IgG and IgM antibodies from the maternal serum to understand the timing of the primary infection. High avidity is suggestive of infection occurring before 3 months.
6. The confirmation of fetal infection is by isolating pathogen specific polymerase chain reaction (PCR) in the amniotic fluid. Amniocentesis should be performed after 18–20 weeks, ideally 6–8 weeks after the detection of primary maternal infection.
7. Fetal infection does not necessarily mean fetal affection, so long term postnatal follow up is needed.
8. Simple preventive measures like hand hygiene, use of vaccines such as for rubella and varicella infections in women of reproductive age would go a long way in reducing maternal and fetal infection.

INTRODUCTION

TORCH is a popular acronym used for congenital infections that can cause significant fetal and neonatal morbidity and mortality. TORCH infections include (TO) xoplasmosis, (R)ubella, (C)ytomegalovirus, and (H)erpes simplex virus. Sometimes the "O" in the acronym is used variably to denote (O)ther agents such as syphilis, varicella zoster virus (VZV), parvovirus B-19, listeriosis, coxsackie virus, hepatitis virus, and zika virus (ZIKV). Transmission of the pathogens may occur in the prenatal, perinatal, and the postnatal period by transplacental route from contact with blood and vaginal secretions or from breast milk. Gestational age of the fetus at the time of infection influences the degree of severity with greater risk of the affection of the fetus, earlier the gestational age. First exposure to these pathogens causes immunity to the mother; however, reinfection can happen with repeated exposure by the same or different strain.

The incidence and prevalence vary in different parts of the world depending on the geographic and socioeconomic condition. The seroprevalence of rubella is 85–90% in childbearing age which means most of the women in the reproductive age group are immune to this infection. A study done in central India evaluated the serological status of IgM and immunoglobulin G (IgG) antibodies in high-risk pregnant women and found that over all TORCH infection (IgM positivity) rate was 61.1%. Rubella was the most prevalent infection (46.5%), followed by herpes simplex virus (HSV) 1 and 2 (41%) and cytomegalovirus (CMV) (34.7%). This study implies the need for proper prenatal counseling and universal immunization which is available for rubella.[1]

ROLE OF SCREENING

Routine screening for TORCH infection is not recommended in national guidelines. However, universal screening for human immunodeficiency virus (HIV), syphilis, and hepatitis B is offered to antenatal women. Few countries have their own guideline regarding TORCH testing; toxoplasmosis is screened routinely in France and Austria because of high prevalence.[2]

INDICATION FOR TORCH TESTING IN PREGNANCY

History and typical clinical presentation of the mother (as in chicken pox), contact with another infected person, travel to endemic areas (ZIKV), or abnormal ultrasound features trigger maternal serological testing for congenital infection.[3] Ultrasound helps in raising suspicion regarding certain congenital infections (toxoplasma, rubella, CMV, herpes simplex, varicella zoster, or ZIKV) and is often the reason to offer serological tests. In case, women present with facial or body rash or ultrasound suggestive of hydrops or fetal anemia, testing for parvovirus should be offered. Ultrasound signs of the affected fetus and clinical presentation of affected neonate suggestive of congenital infection are shown further **(Table 1) (Figs. 1A to K)**.

DIAGNOSIS OF MATERNAL INFECTION

For vertical transmission—maternal infection should occur at time of pregnancy and it should occur for the first time during pregnancy. It is important to order the serology tests correctly, perform the test with the appropriate method, and interpret the report accurately to arrive at a diagnosis.

- *Method:* Enzyme-linked immunosorbent assay (ELISA) tests are most commonly used.
- *How to order serology:*
    - Always paired serology to be ordered which includes both virus-specific antibodies, IgM, and IgG. Ideally, the first sample should be drawn at the time of clinical illness. However, it is not always possible as most infections are asymptomatic. In this scenario, if the prenatal sample taken before the primary infection is available, it can be used to order the serology. Repeat testing of both the antibodies to be ordered after 4 weeks to evaluate the rising or declining trend of the antibody titers. This gives a fair idea about the time of infection in regard to gestational age.
    - Antibody avidity testing also helps in determining the time of infection, the longer the time since the initial infection, the higher the level of avidity.

Maternal serology interpretation ***(Table 2)****:* The appearance and persistence of IgG and IgM antibodies and IgG avidity in different infections over a period of time are shown in **Figures 2 to 4**. High avidity suggests infection has occurred more than 3 months ago.

TABLE 1: Fetal and neonatal signs of different infection.

Infection	Ultrasound features in fetus		Clinical features in affected neonate
	Cranial manifestation	*Extracranial manifestation*	
Toxoplasma	Microcephaly, ventriculomegaly	Hepatosplenomegaly, fetal growth restriction, hyperechogenic bowel, placentomegaly, placental calcifications, oligohydramnios, anhydramnios, and polyhydramnios	Chorioretinitis, anemia, rash, jaundice, pneumonitis, developmental delay, epilepsy, and blindness
Rubella	Microcephaly	Microphthalmia, patent ductus arteriosus (PDA), pulmonary artery stenosis, hepato-splenomegaly, fetal growth restriction, placentomegaly, placental calcifications, oligo-hydramnios/anhydramnios, polyhydramnios	Sensorineural deafness, mental retardation, cataract, retinopathy, chorioretinitis, jaundice, thrombo-cytopenic purpura, meningo-encephalitis, "blueberry muffin rash"
Cytomegalo-virus	Cerebral calcification, periventricular pseud-ocysts, microcephaly, intraventricular synechiae, cerebellar abnormalities (Vermian hypoplasia, cerebellar hemorrhage, calcifications, cysts), malformations of cortical development	Microphthalmia, hepatosplenomegaly, hyperechogenic bowel, hepatic calcification, fetal growth restriction, placentomegaly, placental calcifications, oligohydramnios/ anhydramnios, polyhydramnios	Chorioretinitis, petechiae, skin rash
Herpes simplex	Microcephaly, ventriculomegaly	Micro-ophthalmia, fetal growth restriction, stillbirth, placentomegaly, placental calcifications, oligohydramnios/ anhydramnios, polyhydramnios	Meningoencephalitis, mental retardation, chorioretinitis, scarring or blisters on skin
Parvovirus B19	–	Ascites, pericardial effusion, skin edema, hydrops or fetal anemia (MCA-PSV >1.5 MoM) in absence of maternal atypical antibodies, placentomegaly, polyhydramnios	Hydrops, still birth
Zika virus	Microcephaly, ventriculomegaly, calcification, malformation of cortical development, anomalies of corpus callosum, central arthrogryposis	Microphthalmia, hyperechogenic bowel, ascites, hepatosplenomegaly, hydrops, oligo/ polyhydramnios, placentomegaly, fetal growth restriction	Pyramidal and extrapyramidal motor abnormalities, cataract, coloboma
Varicella zoster virus	Cortical atrophy, microcephaly	Soft-tissue calcification, microphthalmia, polyhydramnios	Chorioretinitis, cataracts, optic atrophy, limb paresis, limb defects and dermatomal skin scarring, encephalitis, seizures and Horner syndrome, spinal cord atrophy

(MCA-PSV: middle cerebral artery peak systolic velocity; MoM: multiples of the median)

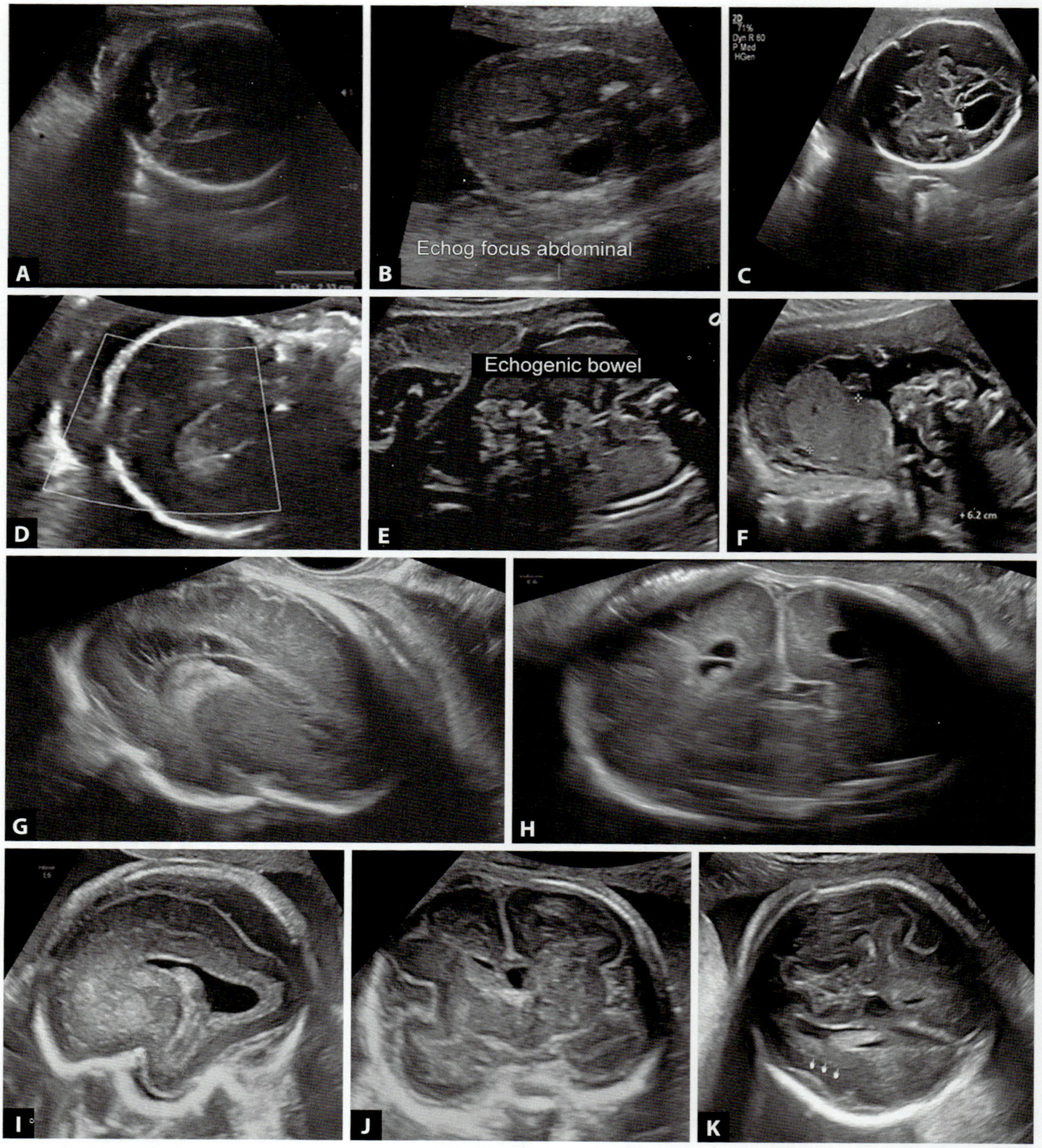

Figs. 1A to K: Ultrasound features suggestive of fetal infection: (A) Dilated cisterna magna; (B) Echogenic foci in liver; (C) Ventriculomegaly; (D) Intracerebral calcifications; (E) Echogenic bowel; (F) Placentomegaly; (G) Periventricular cystic changes; (H) Periventricular cysts; (I to K) Periventricular halo.

Courtesy:

Figures 1A to F: Dr Sumitra Bachani, Delhi.

Figures 1G to K: Dr Seema Yadagiri, Gulbarga, Karnataka.

TABLE 2: Maternal serology interpretation.[4]

IgM	***IgG***	***IgG avidity***	***Interpretation***
Negative	Negative		Susceptible
Positive	Negative		Acute infection*
Negative	Positive		Past infection**
Positive	Positive		Subacute infection***
Positive	Positive	Low avidity	Infection within 3 months
Positive	Positive	High avidity	Infection before 3 months

*To confirm with repeat serology after 4 weeks.
**Avidity helps in deciding time of infection.
***Avidity, detailed history, and ultrasound help in deciding time of infection.

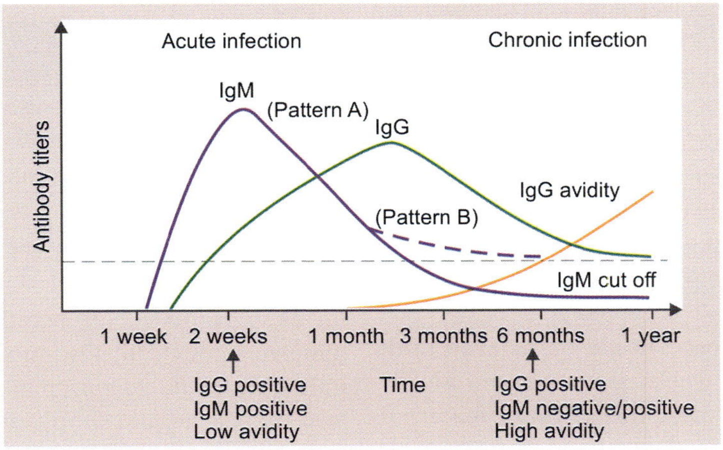

Fig. 2: Toxoplasmosis.[5] (Ig: immunoglobulin)

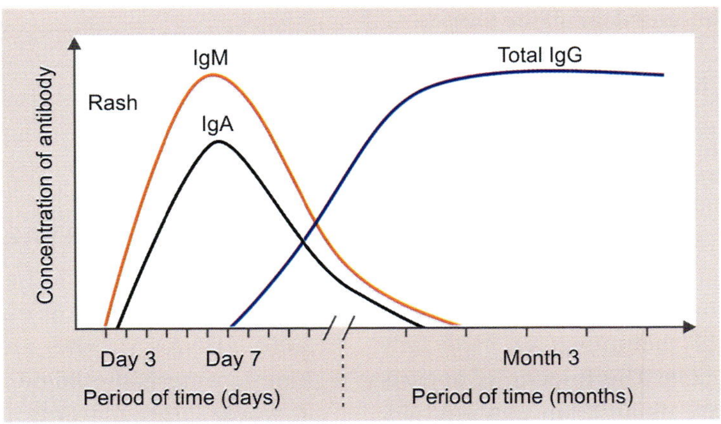

Fig. 3: Rubella.[6] (Ig: immunoglobulin)

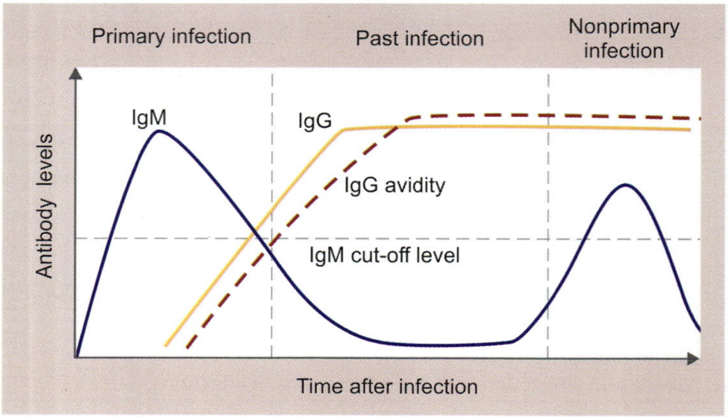

Fig. 4: Cytomegalovirus.[7] (Ig: immunoglobulin)

DIAGNOSIS OF FETAL INFECTION

Regarding diagnosis of fetal infection should be taken into consideration:

- Infection in the early gestation causes a higher chance of affecting the fetus.
- Invasive testing (amniocentesis or cordocentesis) for pathogen-specific PCR test helps in confirmation of fetal infection.
- Amniocentesis should be delayed until after 18–20 weeks' gestation and ideally 6–8 weeks after the primary maternal infection.
- Fetal infection does not necessarily mean fetal affection. So, ultrasound follow-up should be continued for all the fetuses.

SPECIFIC INFECTIONS

Toxoplasmosis

Toxoplasma gondii is a parasite acquired by the ingestion of toxoplasma tissue cysts found in meat or unwashed salads/vegetables, so pregnant women should not consume raw or undercooked meat and wash their hands thoroughly before eating, especially after handling cats. The infectious oocysts are secreted by cats and can contaminate soil. Two thirds of women are found to be asymptomatic on acquiring primary maternal infection; the remainder have a mild coryzal illness with malaise, low-grade fever, headache, and lymphadenopathy.

TABLE 3: Risk of fetal infection with gestational age.[10]

Gestational age	*Risk of fetal infection*	*Risk of fetal affection*
13 weeks	4–15%	61%
26 weeks	44%	25%
36 weeks	>60%	9%

FETAL INFECTION

The overall risk of congenital toxoplasmosis following maternal infection ranges from 20 to 50% without treatment. The risk of vertical transmission increases with gestational age[8,9] **(Table 3)**. The main sequelae of congenital toxoplasma infection are listed in **Table 1**.

DIAGNOSIS OF FETAL INFECTION

- Fetal infection should be diagnosed by detection of toxoplasma deoxyribonucleic acid (DNA) in the amniotic fluid. Amniocentesis should be delayed at least 6 weeks after maternal infection and performed after 18 gestational weeks.

- Women should be informed that the sensitivity of current molecular methods in detecting toxoplasma DNA in the amniotic fluid is ≤90%; false-negative results can occur when the DNA concentration is low.
- Ultrasound follow-up of these fetuses should be done 4 weekly, focusing on brain, ocular, and growth assessment.

Treatment

Spiramycin 1 g tablet taken orally three times daily until the end of the pregnancy, in the absence of confirmed vertical transmission, can be used to prevent vertical transmission after maternal toxoplasma infection during pregnancy and should be initiated without delay (within 3 weeks) following maternal seroconversion. If vertical transmission is confirmed, fetal infection should be treated by spiramycin only for 1 week (1 g tablet three times daily), followed by pyrimethamine (50 mg tablet once daily) plus sulfadiazine (1 g tablet three times daily) plus folinic acid (50 mg weekly) throughout the pregnancy and the infant treated for further 1 year.[11] Long-term follow-up of infants is advisable as only 39% of chorioretinitis cases are diagnosed at birth.[12]

Prevention

Washing hands after handling cats, avoiding contamination of food with cat soil, and thoroughly washing salads/vegetables should be practiced as preventive measures.

Rubella

Rubella (German measles) is a single-stranded ribonucleic acid (RNA) virus of togavirus family that spreads by respiratory droplets.[13] The incubation period is 2–3 weeks and the infectious stage is 7 days before until 10 days after onset of rash. Viremia occurs 7–9 days after exposure. Symptoms are characteristic maculopapular rashes which start from the face, then involve the trunk, lasting for 3 days. This may be accompanied with malaise, fever, headache, conjunctivitis, and occasionally postauricular, suboccipital, and posterior cervical lymphadenopathy. Overt clinical symptoms manifest only in 50–75% women; hence, clinical history may not always suggest prior illness.[14]

Fetal Infection

Rubella is one of the most teratogenic viruses. The risk of fetal infection decreases with increasing gestational age of acquiring maternal infection. Risk of developing congenital rubella syndrome (CRS) is greatest when infection occurs earlier in gestation **(Table 4)**. Reinfection is rare and the chance of CRS is <5%.

The four most common anomalies in CRS are sensorineural deafness, eye defects, central nervous system (CNS) defects, and cardiac defects **(Table 1)**. Gregg's triad is a classical presentation where the baby has microcephaly, patent ductus arteriosus (PDA), and congenital cataract.

Diagnosing Fetal Infection

Infection of the fetus can be confirmed by amniocentesis. This is usually delayed until

TABLE 4: Risk of fetal infection with gestational age.[10]

Gestational age	*Risk of fetal infection*	*Risk of fetal affection (congenital rubella syndrome)*
<12 weeks	90%	97%
12–16 weeks	55%	20%
>16 weeks	45%	Minimal risk of deafness only

after 18–20 weeks' gestation, when fetal urination is established.

- Invasive testing is usually performed for primary maternal infections occurring between 12 and 16 weeks of gestation, the risk of infection to the fetus after that time being small.
- The viral nucleic acid can be detected in the amniotic fluid using PCR; this test has high sensitivity and specificity (87% and 99%, respectively).[15]
- Risk of false-negative result is there if amniocentesis is performed within 6 weeks of the primary maternal infection. A negative result in these circumstances may require repeat invasive testing later.
- Primary infection before 12 weeks' gestation carries very high risk of an infected fetus developing severe abnormalities. Termination of pregnancy even without invasive testing can be considered in this situation.[3]

Prevention

Although being the most teratogenic virus, rubella infection can be preventable with vaccination. The trivalent measles, mumps, and rubella (MMR) vaccine is a part of the National Immunization Program. It should be administered to all children between 12 and 15 months and second dose to be administered at least 1 month after first dose but before 6 years. It gives long-term immunity in 95% of individuals. Susceptible adolescent girls and all women of reproductive age group should receive vaccine (RA 27/3 vaccine, subcutaneously, 0.5 mL). Pregnancy should be deferred for 1 month after the vaccine.[16] However, termination is not advised in cases of conception within a month as no adverse outcome is reported on follow-up studies. Susceptible pregnant women should be offered vaccination immediately after delivery.

Cytomegalovirus

Cytomegalovirus is the most common viral cause of congenital infection, affecting 0.2–2.2% of all live births.[17] It is the leading nongenetic cause of sensorineural hearing loss (SNHL) and a major cause of neurological disability. Around 10–15% of neonates with congenital CMV will be symptomatic at birth and up to 25% of infected children have long-term sequelae.[18] The maternal infection is usually asymptomatic, but a minority may experience symptoms like those of infectious mononucleosis (glandular fever) such as fever, malaise, myalgia, cervical lymphadenopathy, and less commonly, hepatitis and pneumonia, though few suffer long-term sequelae. Women who gave birth in <3 years before a new pregnancy and whose infant is school going or in childcare have 7% risk of getting an infection in the first trimester.[19]

Cytomegalovirus infection may be primary which is more common and acquired for the first time during pregnancy or nonprimary infection which may result from reactivation of prior infection or reinfection with a different strain of the virus. Primary CMV infections during pregnancy have a 30–40% risk of congenital infection, as compared to 1–2% following a nonprimary infection.[20,21] Timing of maternal CMV infection affects risk of mother-to-child transmission and congenital CMV severity **(Table 5)**.[22]

Similarly, neonates are more symptomatic when maternal infection happens earlier, 9.1% in the first, 0.3% in the second, and 0.4% in the third trimester of pregnancy. Earlier study showed nearly similar risk of congenital infection with respect to the period of gestation at which primary infection occurs, increasing from around 30% in the first trimester to 47% in the third trimester.[23]

TABLE 5: Risk of fetal infection with gestational age.[22]

Gestational age	*Risk of fetal infection*	*Risk of fetal affection*	*Risk of sensorineural hearing loss*
First trimester	36.8%	19.3%	22.8%
Second trimester	40.3%	0.9%	0.1%
Third trimester	66.2%	0.4%	0%

Fetal Infection

Detectable ultrasound features and congenital infection is described in **Table 1**.

Diagnosis of Fetal Infection

- Detection of CMV DNA on PCR analysis of the amniotic fluid is diagnostic.
- Amniocentesis should be delayed until at least 8 weeks after estimated time of maternal infection and after 20 gestational weeks.[3]
- The most common cause for false-negative results is the time interval between infection and amniocentesis of <8 weeks and gestational age at amniocentesis of <18 weeks.[3]
- Congenital CMV should be confirmed at birth following an antenatal diagnosis of maternal infection, even when a diagnosis of fetal infection has been made by invasive sampling, using infant's urine sample or saliva swab for CMV-PCR as soon as possible after birth and it is important to collect samples within 3 weeks of birth to confirm congenital rather than postnatal acquisition of CMV.

Prevention

Due to the lack of randomized controlled trials, high-dose valacyclovir for congenital CMV infection should only be given in the context of research. Similarly, CMV-specific hyperimmune globulin (HIG) although showed promising results in symptomatic infections in few studies, the recommendation is to not to be used in treatment of congenital CMV infection.[3] There is currently no licensed vaccine for CMV.

Prenatal education on strategies to reduce risk is effective.[24] Emphasis on avoiding exposure to younger children's bodily fluids, avoiding sharing foods, drinks, utensils, kissing on the lips, washing hands thoroughly after being in contact with saliva, nose drippings, or urine of young children.[25]

Herpes Simplex Virus

Herpes simplex virus is a double-stranded DNA virus belonging to the Alphaherpesvirinae family. Infection in pregnancy can be caused by two types: HSV 1 which is responsible mainly for herpes labialis, gingivostomatitis, and keratoconjunctivitis, while HSV 2 is the primary etiologic agent of genital herpes. Cervix and urethra are involved in 80%. It occurs mainly by sexual contact and also by contact with mucosa or abraded skin. The maternal infection can be primary, nonprimary, or recurrent.

Vertical transmission occurs mainly during delivery resulting in neonatal herpes, followed by postpartum transmission by contact with mother, healthcare worker, or family member. Transplacental transmission rarely occurs (5%). When the mother has primary infection and the seroconversion occurs prior to 30–34 weeks, the risk of transmission is 20–25%, but in nonprimary or recurrent infection, the overall risk of transmission is <1%. In a primary herpes infection, when genital lesions are present at the time of delivery and the baby is delivered vaginally, the risk of neonatal herpes is estimated to be 41%.[26]

Those with suspicion of infection can undergo testing by two basic modalities: (1) Viral detection techniques and (2) antibody detection techniques. Those presenting with genital ulcers or mucocutaneous lesions are subjected to HSV detection by PCR technique (sensitivity 96–98%) and cultures (sensitivity 80% for primary lesions and 40% for secondary lesions). As most primary infections can be asymptomatic, hence, serology should also be done in all cases suspected to be HSV as it may be a nonprimary, recurrent, or asymptomatic primary case. The sensitivity of ELISA for HSV 1 and 2 antibody testing is 90–100%.[27]

Fetal Infection

Infection during first or second trimester is not associated with increased risk of miscarriage or congenital anomaly; in third trimester, it can cause fetal affection **(Table 1)**. Neonatal herpes is caused by HSV 1 in 50% cases and rest by HSV 2. Neonatal HSV infections can be classified as disseminated disease (25%); CNS disease (30%); and disease limited to the skin, eyes, or mouth (45%). Mortality is highest for disseminated disease (30%) and lowest for local lesions and long-term neurological sequelae is noted in 20% of survivors.[28]

Prevention

Safe sexual practice is the only way to prevent viral exposure to the mother. When there is active lesion seen at the time of delivery, cesarean section is advised to prevent fetal infection.

Treatment

Acyclovir is used as an antiviral medication in active herpes infection. Orally, 400 mg three times a day is given for 7–10 days. To prevent recurrence at term, suppressive therapy is offered from 36 weeks until delivery, 400 mg orally three times a day.[29]

Parvovirus B19

Parvovirus B19 is a single-stranded DNA, nonenveloped virus from the family *Parvoviridae*. It causes a common childhood viral infection (fifth disease). About 60–75% of pregnant women are immune to parvovirus infection. Infected children exhibit a characteristic facial rash and fever, which is known as "slapped-cheek syndrome" which often runs in epidemics. It is spread by respiratory droplets from infected people, by blood or blood-product transfusion or by transplacental passage.

The most common trigger for maternal testing for parvovirus B19 in pregnancy is a report of recent exposure; it can also result from an incidental finding of fetal hydrops on ultrasound. When a mother contracts infection, the risk of vertical transmission to the fetus ranges from 25 to 32%.[30] Serial ultrasound monitoring, for evidence of ascites, cardiomegaly, hydrops fetalis, and raised middle cerebral artery peak systolic velocity (MCA-PSV), should start 4 weeks after infection or seroconversion and be performed every 1–2 weeks thereafter until 12 weeks after infection[3] **(Figs. 5A to C)**. Intrauterine red blood cell transfusion (IUBT) can be used to treat fetal hydrops caused by parvovirus B19. The anemia resolves after 6 weeks of infection and one or two IUBT are sufficient. Cerebral imaging should also be considered for potential long-term neurodevelopmental sequelae.

Zika Virus

Zika virus is a flavivirus that is usually transmitted by *Aedes* mosquitoes, but it can also be transmitted from human to human

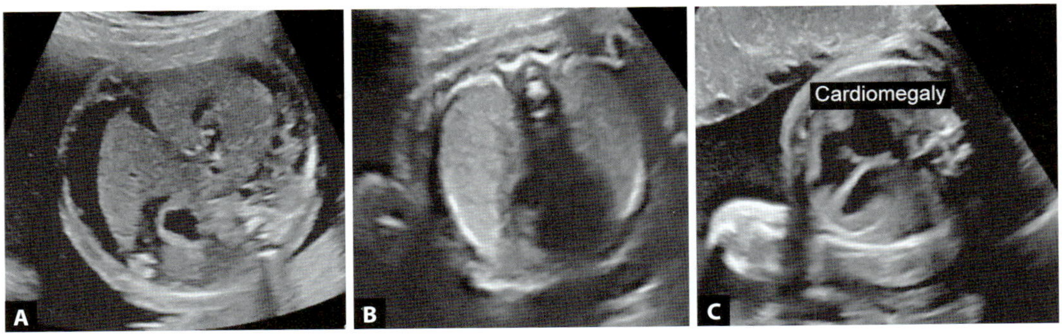

Figs. 5A to C: (A) Ascites; (B) Pleural effusion; (C) Cardiomegaly.
Courtesy: Dr Sumitra Bachani, Delhi.

through sexual contact. The World Health Organization (WHO) advised that pregnant women avoid travel to ZIKV-affected areas and should practice safe sex or abstinence for 6 months after their return from affected areas.[31] Pregnant women with suggestive symptoms and a history of recent travel to ZIKV-affected area, or of sexual contact with a person returning from an affected area, should be investigated for ZIKV.[3]

It is usually a mild self-limiting illness and the primary test is real-time reverse transcription-PCR (rRT-PCR) of serum and urine. The value of amniocentesis to diagnose fetal infection is limited. A baseline fetal ultrasound examination should be performed after potential maternal exposure and repeated in third trimester. ZIKV infection causes brain abnormalities such as microcephaly **(Table 1)**. Also, risk of congenital disabilities is higher with earlier infection and independent of maternal symptoms. Currently, no effective treatment and vaccine are available; only preventive measures are effective.

Varicella Zoster Virus

Varicella zoster virus is a DNA virus of the herpesvirus family that is highly contagious. Primary infection in pregnancy occurs in only 3 per 1,000 pregnancies.

TABLE 6: Risk of fetal infection with gestational age.[3]

Gestational age	*Risk of fetal infection*
13 weeks	0.5%
13–20 weeks	2%
>20 weeks	No risk

Varicella (chickenpox) has a characteristic maculopapular rash, which later becomes vesicular and subsequently crust over to heal completely. This is accompanied by fever and malaise. Over 90% antenatal women are immune due to childhood infection. Pregnant women developing herpes zoster (shingles, caused by the same virus) during pregnancy do not cause fetal infection. The risk of fetal infection in relation to gestational age is shown in **Table 6**. There is a 25% risk of clinical neonatal varicella if infection occurs after 36 weeks.[3] Following maternal infection in the first 20 gestational weeks, serial ultrasound examinations should be performed from 5 weeks after the initial infection or from 16 gestational weeks, whichever is earlier. Following exposure to VZV, nonimmune pregnant women should be offered varicella zoster immunoglobulin (VZIG) within 10 days after exposure. Oral acyclovir can also be considered as postexposure prophylaxis from 7 days after exposure.[3]

REFERENCES

1. Manjunathachar HV, Singh KN, Chouksey V, Kumar R, Sharma RK, Barde PV. Prevalence of torch infections and its associated poor outcome in high-risk pregnant women of Central India: Time to think for prevention strategies. Indian J Med Microbiol. 2020;38(3 & 4):379-84.
2. Prusa AR, Kasper DC, Pollak A, Gleiss A, Waldhoer T, Hayde M. The Austrian Toxoplasmosis Register, 1992-2008. Clin Infect Dis. 2015;60(2):e4-10.
3. Khalil A, Sotiriadis A, Chaoui R, da Silva Costa F, D'Antonio F, Heath PT, et al. ISUOG Practice Guidelines: role of ultrasound in congenital infection. Ultrasound Obstet Gynecol. 2020;56(1):128-51.
4. FOGSI. (2014). Screening and management of TORCH in pregnancy. [online] Available from https://www-fogsi-org.webpkgcache.com/doc/-/s/www.fogsi.org/wp-content/uploads/2015/11/smtp.pdf [Last accessed March, 2024].
5. Teimouri A, Mohtasebi S, Kazemirad E, Keshavarz H. Role of Toxoplasma gondii IgG Avidity Testing in Discriminating between Acute and Chronic Toxoplasmosis in Pregnancy. J Clin Microbiol. 2020;58(9): e00505-20.
6. Dimech W, Grangeot-Keros L, Vauloup-Fellous C. Standardization of Assays That Detect Anti-Rubella Virus IgG Antibodies. Clin Microbiol Rev. 2016;29(1):163-74.
7. Iijima S. Pitfalls in the Serological Evaluation of Maternal Cytomegalovirus Infection as a Potential Cause of Fetal and Neonatal Involvements: A Narrative Literature Review. J Clin Med. 2022;11(17):5006.
8. Dunn D, Wallon M, Peyron F, Petersen E, Peckham C, Gilbert R. Mother-to-child transmission of toxoplasmosis: risk estimates for clinical counseling. Lancet. 1999;353:1829-33.
9. Desmonts G, Couvreur J. Congenital toxoplasmosis. Prospective study of the outcome of pregnancy in 542 women with toxoplasmosis acquired during pregnancy. Ann Pediatr (Paris). 1984;31:805-9.
10. Sharma KA, Deka D. TORCH Infections in Pregnancy. In: Trivedi SS, Puri M, Agrawal S (Eds). Management of High-Risk Pregnancy: A Practical Approach, 3rd edition. New Delhi: Jaypee Brothers Medical Publishers (P) Ltd.; 2022. pp. 347-55.
11. Stray-Pedersen B. Treatment of toxoplasmosis in the pregnant mother and newborn child. Scand J Infect Dis Suppl. 1992;84:23-31.
12. Berrébi A, Assouline C, Bessières MH, Lathière M, Cassaing S, Minville V, et al. Long-term outcome of children with congenital toxoplasmosis. Am J Obstet Gynecol. 2010;203(6):552.e1-6.
13. Gershon AA. Rubella virus (German Measles). In: John E, Bennett RD, Blaser MJ (Eds). Mandell, Douglas, and Bennett's Principles and Practice of Infectious Diseases, 8th edition. Amsterdam, The Netherlands: Elsevier Health Sciences; 2014.
14. Cochi SL, Edmonds LE, Dyer K, Greaves WL, Marks JS, Rovira EZ, et al. Congenital rubella syndrome in the United States, 1970-1985. On the verge of elimination. Am J Epidemiol. 1989;129(2):349-61.
15. Macé M, Cointe D, Six C, Levy-Bruhl D, Parent du Châtelet I, Ingrand D, et al. Diagnostic value of reverse transcription-PCR of amniotic fluid for prenatal diagnosis of congenital rubella infection in pregnant women with confirmed primary rubella infection. J Clin Microbiol. 2004;42(10):4818-20.
16. CDC. (2020). Pregnancy and Rubella. [online] Available from https://www.cdc.gov/rubella/pregnancy.html [Last accessed March, 2024].
17. Dollard SC, Grosse SD, Ross DS. New estimates of the prevalence of neurological and sensory sequelae and mortality associated with congenital cytomegalovirus infection. Rev Med Virol. 2007;17(5):355-63.
18. Townsend CL, Forsgren M, Ahlfors K, Ivarsson SA, Tookey PA, Peckham CS. Long-term Outcomes of Congenital Cytomegalovirus Infection in Sweden and the United Kingdom. Clin Infect Dis. 2013;56(9):1232-9.

19. Leruez-Ville M, Guilleminot T, Stirnemann J, Salomon LJ, Spaggiari E, Faure-Bardon V, et al. Quantifying the Burden of Congenital Cytomegalovirus Infection With Long-term Sequelae in Subsequent Pregnancies of Women Seronegative at Their First Pregnancy. Clin Infect Dis. 2020;71(7):1598-603.
20. Fowler KB, Stagno S, Pass RF, Britt WJ, Boll TJ, Alford CA. The outcome of congenital CMV infection in relation to maternal antibody status. N Engl J Med. 1992;326:663-7.
21. Kenneson A, Cannon MJ. Review and meta-analysis of the epidemiology of congenital CMV infection. Rev Med Virol. 2009;17:253-76.
22. Chatzakis C, Ville Y, Makrydimas G, Dinas K, Zavlanos A, Sotiriadis A. Timing of primary maternal cytomegalovirus infection and rates of vertical transmission and fetal consequences. Am J Obstet Gynecol. 2020;223(6):870-83.e11.
23. Enders G, Daiminger A, Bäder U, Exler S, Enders M. Intrauterine transmission and clinical outcome of 248 pregnancies with primary cytomegalovirus infection in relation to gestational age. J Clin Virol. 2011;52(3):244-6.
24. Pesch MH, Saunders NA, Abdelnabi S. Cytomegalovirus Infection in Pregnancy: Prevention, Presentation, Management and Neonatal Outcomes. J Midwifery Womens Health. 2021;66(3):397-402.
25. Rawlinson WD, Boppana SB, Fowler KB, Kimberlin DW, Lazzarotto T, Alain S, et al. Congenital cytomegalovirus infection in pregnancy and the neonate: consensus recommendations for prevention, diagnosis, and therapy. Lancet Infect Dis. 2017;17:e177-88.
26. RCOG. Management of genital herpes in pregnancy. [online] Available from https://www.rcog.org.uk/guidance/browse-all-guidance/other-guidelines-and-reports/management-of-genital-herpes-in-pregnancy/ [Last accessed March, 2024].
27. Moseley RC, Corey L, Benjamin D, Winter C, Remington ML. Comparison of viral isolation, direct immunofluorescence, and indirect immunoperoxidase techniques for detection of genital herpes simplex virus infection. J Clin Microbiol. 1981;13:913-8.
28. British Paediatric Surveillance Unit. BPSU 21st Annual Report 2006-2007. London: British Paediatric Surveillance Unit/Royal College of Paediatrics and Child Health; 2007.
29. Management of Genital Herpes in Pregnancy: ACOG Practice Bulletin Summary, Number 220. Obstet Gynecol. 2020;135(5):1236-8.
30. Puccetti C, Contoli M, Bonvicini F, Cervi F, Simonazzi G, Gallinella G, et al. Parvovirus B19 in pregnancy: possible consequences of vertical transmission. Prenat Diagn. 2012;32(9):897-902.
31. WHO. (2016). Vector control operations framework for Zika virus. https://www.who.int/publications/i/item/WHO-ZIKV-VC-16.4 [Last accessed March, 2024].

CHAPTER 12

Rh-negative Pregnancy and Immune Hydrops

Sumitra Bachani, Noopur Chawla Pruthi, Aprajita Gupta, Poornima Sharma

KEY POINTS

This chapter comprehensively addresses rhesus (Rh)-negative pregnancy, elucidating the risks of alloimmunization and its complications of fetal anemia, neonatal jaundice, and hydrops fetalis.

1. The importance of screening at booking to identify Rh-negative women should be emphasized and the risk of sensitization should be assessed.
2. If the pregnancy is found to be at risk, routine anti-D prophylaxis should be given at 28 weeks and then within 72 hours of delivery if indirect Coombs test (ICT) is found to be negative and the baby is D-positive, respectively. Therefore, patient education regarding these risks and the significance of anti-D prophylaxis is paramount.
3. All isoimmunized pregnancies, where critical titers have reached, are monitored with middle cerebral artery peak systolic velocity (MCA PSV) Doppler as a crucial tool for monitoring fetal anemia.
4. Intrauterine transfusion (IUT) with blood type O and D-negative packed red cells to the fetus via the umbilical vein is started when MCA PSV is beyond 1.5 multiple of median (MoM).
5. Additionally, the chapter underscores the importance of intravenous immunoglobulin (IVIG) therapy in delaying the need for IUT.
6. Referral to fetal medicine specialists for high-risk cases ensures timely intervention and comprehensive management, ultimately optimizing maternal and fetal outcomes in Rh-negative pregnancies.

INTRODUCTION

One of the major blood group systems the ABO includes the surface antigens A, B, and Rh antigen D present on the human erythrocytes. The Rh blood group antigens comprises the CDE system which includes five major erythrocyte antigens: C, c, D, E, and e.[1] An individual who lacks a specific erythrocyte antigen may produce antibodies against it when exposed to that antigen. Some of these antigens are immunologically relevant. In an antenatal woman, if these antibodies are present, they can cross the placental barrier and react with fetal red cells that contain the associated antigens, resulting in fetal anemia, hydrops fetalis, and ultimately death in utero or severe neonatal jaundice and mortality.[1]

The prevalence of red cell alloimmunization in pregnancy is about 1%. The risk of fetal anemia is greatest with anti-D, -c, and -K antibodies. Other antibodies that potentially cause significant fetal anemia include anti-E, -Fya, -Jka, -C, and -Ce. There are numerous other antibodies that usually only cause mild hemolysis.[2] Most cases of severe fetal anemia requiring antenatal transfusion are attributable to anti-D, anti-Kell, anti-c, or anti-E alloimmunization.[1]

The most common cause of hemolytic disease of newborn is actually ABO blood group incompatibility, but the resultant anemia is usually mild. About 20% of all infants have an ABO incompatibility, but only 5% are clinically affected. The ABO incompatibility causes rapid clearance of fetal red cells before they elicit an immune response, thus causing a reduction in Rh alloimmunization.[1]

MECHANISM OF ALLOIMMUNIZATION

When an Rh-negative woman bears a Rh-positive fetus, the pregnancy is at a risk of iso- or alloimmunization. The fetal red cells containing the Rh antigen enter the maternal circulation, i.e., fetomaternal hemorrhage (FMH). As less as 0.1 mL of fetal erythrocytes are sufficient to sensitize the D-negative mother.[1] FMH can occur throughout pregnancy, incidence being 5% in the first trimester, up to 46% in third trimester, and maximum 49% at the time of delivery. There can be few sensitizing events which also lead to FMH **(Box 1)**.

Fetal erythrocytes elicit an anamnestic immune response from the maternal circulation which leads to the formation of two types of antibodies: Immunoglobulin M (IgM) and IgG. The primary response involves clearance of the Rh antigen by macrophages; processed and transferred to plasma stem cell precursors (develop an almost permanent immunologic memory) IgM, the first antibody to appear in the maternal circulation cannot cross the placental barrier as it is a larger molecule and therefore is not harmful to the fetus. With subsequent exposure, the plasma cell line proliferates to produce humoral antibodies, the secondary immune response.

BOX 1: Precursors for fetomaternal hemorrhage.[1]

- *Pregnancy loss:* Abortion (spontaneous or elective), ectopic pregnancy, fetal death (any trimester)
- *Procedures:* Amniocentesis, chorionic villous sampling, fetal blood sampling, molar pregnancy evacuation
- *Others:*
  - Antepartum bleeding (including threatened abortion)
  - Delivery (vaginal/cesarean)
  - External cephalic version
  - Placental abruption, manual removal of placenta
  - Trauma to the abdomen during pregnancy

Immunoglobulin G, also called incomplete or blocking antibody, is a small molecule that can cross the placental barrier and cause fetal red cell hemolysis. As it appears much later than IgM antibody, the first pregnancy in Rh-negative women is not affected.[1]

If the woman is D-negative, but the husband is D-positive, IgG titers in maternal serum are assessed using the ICT at the booking visit. A sample of the mother's blood is taken and tested for antibodies by serial dilution. If the antibodies are absent, the ICT test is considered negative. ICT is positive in alloimmunized pregnancy and antibody titer at which significant fetal anemia may develop is called the critical titer. A titer ≥1:16 (tube method) or ≥1:32 (gel method) indicates the possibility of severe hemolytic disease.[1] One must confirm from the laboratory which method has been used for the test.

The spectrum of hemolytic disease of newborn includes:

- Hydrops fetalis
- Icterus gravis neonatorum
- Congenital anemia of newborn

Hydrops fetalis: This is the most severe manifestation of Rh hemolytic disease, characterized by severe fetal anemia, tissue hypoxemia, and metabolic acidosis. Fetal hydrops is diagnosed when fluid accumulates in two or more body cavities, such as ascites, pleural effusion, pericardial effusion, or skin edema seen on ultrasonography. Polyhydramnios may also be present. Perinatal survival rates, even with treatment, have been reported at 84%, with hydropic fetuses exhibiting lower survival rates (74%) compared to nonhydropic fetuses (94%) **(Fig. 1)**.[2]

Icterus gravis neonatorum: The circulating antibodies lyse the fetal erythrocytes which leads to an increase in unconjugated bilirubin. During the in utero life, this unconjugated bilirubin is filtered by the placenta. After delivery, the neonatal liver cannot handle a large load of bilirubin and thus, the baby starts showing the symptoms and signs of jaundice within the first 24 hours of life. If the levels are critical, bilirubin crosses the blood–brain barrier and causes damage to the basal ganglia, causing manifestations of kernicterus and cerebral palsy.

Congenital anemia of the newborn: This is the mildest form of the disease and usually appears in the first few weeks of life. The hemolysis is seen up to 6 weeks after which the antibodies disappear. This is associated with hepatosplenomegaly in the neonate due to compensatory erythropoiesis in these organs.

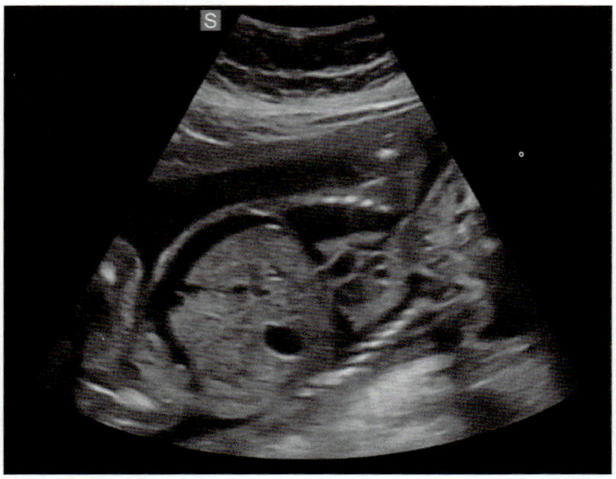

Fig. 1: Ultrasonographic (USG) image of a hydropic fetus at 29 weeks.

PREVENTION OF Rh ALLOIMMUNIZATION[1]

In regions lacking routine antenatal anti-D prophylaxis (RAADP), approximately 10% of D-negative pregnancies become alloimmunized. To mitigate this risk, routine anti-D prophylaxis is administered to all D-negative, nonsensitized (ICT-negative) women at 28 weeks of gestation, resulting in a significant reduction of the third-trimester alloimmunization rate to 0.1% **(Table 1)**.

The standard intramuscular dose of anti-D immunoglobulin, which is 300 µg or 1,500 IU, protects against FMH of up to 30 mL of whole blood or 15 mL of red cells. Newborns of D-negative mothers are also D-negative in 40% cases; administration of immunoglobulin is recommended only after confirming the newborn to be D-positive. In cases of uncertainty regarding the need of anti-D immunoglobulin, it is advisable to administer. It acts by coating the Rh antigen on the fetal erythrocytes following which they are removed from the maternal circulation primarily by the spleen. These coated erythrocytes also block further production of IgG from the B cells.

Traditionally, anti-D is manufactured by fractionating IgG from pooled plasma obtained from donors, predominantly Rh disease-(RhD)-negative men who have been

TABLE 1: Risk of alloimmunization.

Pregnancy	*Percentage of alloimmunization*
First rhesus (Rh) incompatible pregnancy untreated with ABO compatible	16%
With ABO incompatible	2%
Postpartum anti-D prophylaxis	1–2%
Antepartum + postpartum anti-D prophylaxis	0.1–0.2%

intentionally immunized with RhD-positive red blood cells (RBCs). The resulting IgG is polyclonal and known as polyclonal anti-D (poly anti-D). However, this method has several drawbacks, including the necessity for human donors, restricted production capacity, potential risk of viral transmission, and intermittent shortages. To address these limitations, monoclonal anti-D (mono anti-D) was introduced. Mono anti-D is produced using the hybridoma technique, which has largely mitigated the issues associated with poly anti-D production. The manufacturer of mono anti-D utilized recombinant deoxyribonucleic acid (DNA) technology to develop anti-D IgG antibodies **(Fig. 2)**. These antibodies were derived from the genes for anti-D obtained from the hybridoma. The genes encoding the antibody from this hybridoma were isolated and introduced into Chinese hamster ovarian (CHO) cells. This allowed the cells to express recombinant anti-D (R-anti-D).[3]

An ICT is recommended at 28 weeks for identifying women who have become alloimmunized prior to administering RAADP. If it is inadvertently missed after delivery, it should be given as soon as

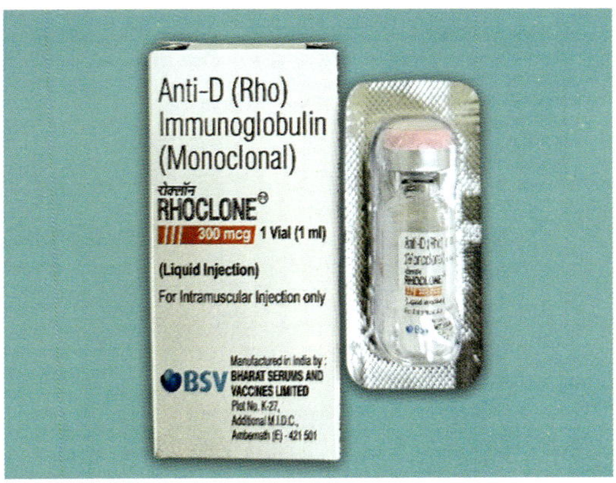

Fig. 2: Monoclonal anti-D injection developed from recombinant deoxyribonucleic acid (DNA) technology.

possible, as some protection is still offered for up to 28 days postpartum. The half-life of anti-D immunoglobulin ranges from 16 to 24 days, which is why it is administered both in the third trimester and following delivery.

Furthermore, anti-D immunoglobulin is administered following pregnancy-related events that could potentially result in sensitization **(Table 2)**. Anti-D immunoglobulin may result in a weakly positive (1:1–1:4) ICT titer in the mother. It is important, however, that neither ICT should be done after administering RAADP nor this result should not be mistaken for the development of alloimmunization.[1]

In cases of severe antepartum or postpartum hemorrhage, abdominal trauma, and manual removal of placenta, the Kleihauer–Betke (KB) test can be utilized to estimate the optimal dosage required in such situations as the FMH will be higher than 30 mL.[8] It is an acid elution test; on addition of citric acid phosphate buffer, maternal red cells become colorless and have ghost appearance, while fetal RBCs retain their color. The number of fetal RBC per 1,000 maternal ghost cells are counted. An alternative approach to quantifying FMH involves flow cytometry, which utilizes monoclonal antibodies specific to hemoglobin F or the D antigen and measures the resulting fluorescence intensity. While flow cytometry has been reported to offer higher sensitivity and accuracy compared to the KB test, it requires specialized technology that is not commonly available in many hospitals.

Fetomaternal Hemorrhage by Kleihauer–Betke Test

Amount of bleed (FMH) = Number of fetal cells/1,000 adult cells × 5,000 (maternal blood volume)

TABLE 2: Recommendations by various organizations for the use of anti-D immunoprophylaxis during pregnancy.[4-7]

Event timeline (weeks = w)	*Sensitization incidence*	*ACOG*	*RCOG*	*FOGSI*	*WHO*
Routine prophylaxis		*At 28 w:* A single antenatal dose of 300 µg followed by a second dose after birth	Two injections (100 µg at 28 and 34 w each) or as a single 300 µg administration at 28 w and after delivery	*At 28 w:* Single antenatal dose of 300 µg followed by a second dose after birth	
Spontaneous miscarriage ≤12 w	1.5–2%	50 µg	Not indicated, unless associated with heavy/ repeated bleeding or with abdominal pain	• *≤20 w:* 150 µg • *>20 w:* 300 µg	Not recommended
Surgical or medical termination of pregnancy	4–5%	• 50 µg (before 12 w) • 300 µg (after 12 w)	• *<12 w:* 50 µg • *12–20 w:* 50 µg • *After 20 w:* 100 µg minimum dose	• *≤20 w:* 150 µg • *>20 w:* 300 µg	• *<12 w:* Not recommended • *≥12 w:* Follow standard of care
Ectopic pregnancy (medically or surgically managed)	Up to 24%	• 50 µg (before 12 w) • 300 µg (after 12 w)	• *<12 w:* 50 µg • *12–20 w:* 50 µg • *After 20 w:* 100 µg minimum dose	• *≤20 w:* 150 µg • *>20 w:* 300 µg	
Invasive procedures such as CVS, amniocentesis, any other sensitizing event		• 50 µg (before 12 w) • 300 µg (after 12 w)	• *12–20 w:* 50 µg • *After 20 w:* 100 µg minimum dose	• *≤20 w:* 150 µg • *>20 w:* 300 µg	
Molar pregnancy		• 50 µg (before 12 w) • 300 µg (after 12 w)	• *<12 w:* 50 µg *12–20 w:* 50 µg • *After 20 w:* 100 µg minimum dose	• *≤20 w:* 150 µg • *>20 w:* 300 µg	

(ACOG: American College of Obstetricians and Gynecologists; CVS: chorionic villus sampling; FOGSI: Federation of Obstetric and Gynaecological Societies of India; RCOG: Royal College of Obstetricians and Gynaecologists; WHO: World Health Organization)

$$\text{Total vials required} = \frac{\text{FMH}}{30^*}$$

*1 vial has 300 µg which neutralizes 30 mL FMH

It should be administered in the deltoid region or anterolateral thigh and gluteal area should be avoided as due to excess fat accumulation during pregnancy, there will be impaired absorption of the drug from that area. A maximum of five vials can be administered in 24 hours. In case a larger dose is required, it can be given intravenous; however, the risk of anaphylaxis is very high.

MANAGEMENT OF WOMEN WITH Rh-NEGATIVE PREGNANCIES

If on booking visit, an antenatal woman tests D-negative and husband is D-positive, there are various methods for ascertaining the risk to this pregnancy. The genotype of the husband can be tested to know if it is homozygous (100% at risk pregnancy) or heterozygous (50% risk). The fetal blood type can be ascertained using the cell-free fetal DNA (noninvasive prenatal test) method to know if the fetus is D-positive or negative. However, these are not cost-effective and very few laboratories are standardized for these tests. Hence, universally, an ICT is done to ascertain if the pregnancy is alloimmunized. If the mother is not alloimmunized at 28 weeks or beyond, anti-D prophylaxis is administered.

If the ICT is positive at booking visit, antibody titers are repeated every 4 weeks till 28 weeks and then fortnightly till delivery or till critical titers reach whichever is earlier. If antibody levels reach the critical titers, there is risk of fetal hemolysis. Earlier method of amniotic fluid spectrophotometry for determining the degree of fetal anemia is now redundant. Studies have established fetal MCA Doppler to positively correlate with the fetal hematocrit.[9]

Estimation of Middle Cerebral Artery Peak Systolic Velocity

During pregnancy, the anemic fetus redirects blood flow to the brain to maintain adequate oxygen levels. This results in an increase in blood velocity due to heightened cardiac output and reduced blood viscosity which can be measured in terms of the MCA PSV. The vessel is interrogated close to its origin from the circle of Willis. The artery closer to the probe is identified and the Doppler gate is placed at an angle of insonation closer to 0°. The PSV is further quantified in terms on MoM values as per the gestational age **(Fig. 3)**.

The threshold of 1.5 MoM for gestational age effectively detects all fetuses with moderate or severe anemia, achieving a sensitivity of 100% and has a false-positive rate of 12%.[1] Surveillance for fetal well-being should be undertaken at a stage of pregnancy, where fetal blood sampling or IUT can be feasibly performed, typically around 18–20 weeks of gestation. From 24 weeks onward, MCA PSV is done every fortnightly if there is no fetal anemia (1 MoM) and weekly once abnormal ultrasound findings suggestive of developing anemia are detected. With worsening MCA PSV, the monitoring is more frequent (twice or thrice a week).[10] Should the MCA PSV surpass 1.5 MoM or if hydrops emerge with anemia being the primary cause, the option of fetal blood sampling and IUT should be contemplated **(Flowchart 1)**.

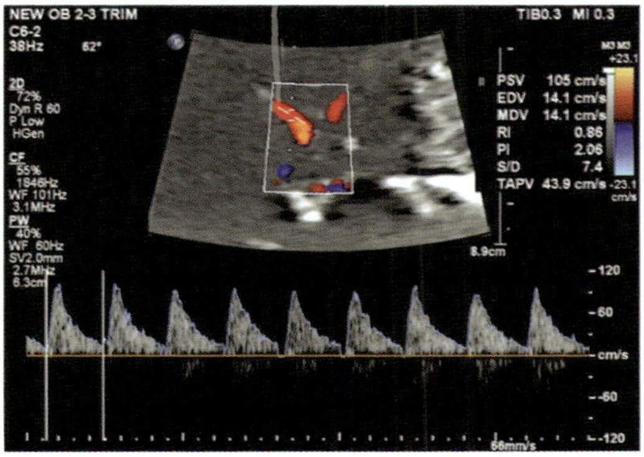

Fig. 3: MCA PSV assessment. (EDV: end-diastolic velocity; MCA: middle cerebral artery; MDV: mean diastolic velocity; PI: pulsatility index; PSV: peak systolic velocity; RI: resistive index; TAPV: timed averaged peak velocity)

Flowchart 1: Management of D-negative pregnancy.[10]

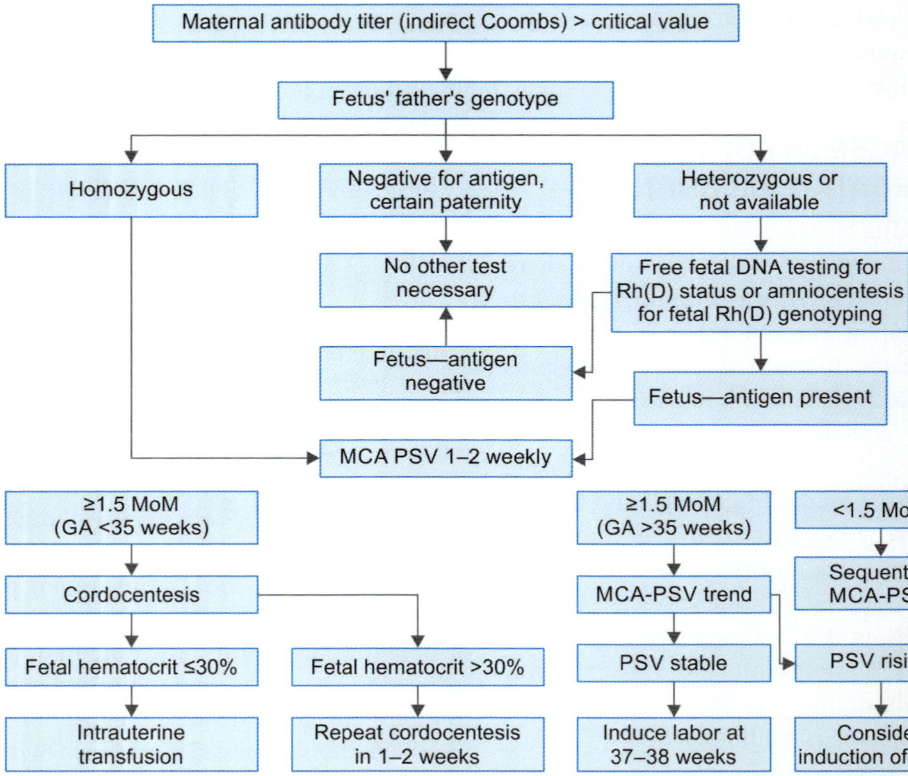

(DNA: deoxyribonucleic acid; GA: gestational age; MCA: middle cerebral artery; MoM: multiple of median; PSV: peak systolic velocity; Rh(D): rhesus disease)

After 34 weeks of gestation, there is a notable rise in the false-positive rate of MCA PSV. This increase is linked to the inherent increase in cardiac output that typically occurs during this late stage of pregnancy, hence this modality is not reliable.[1]

INTRAUTERINE TRANSFUSION

Generally, fetal transfusion procedures are undertaken up to the 34th–35th week of gestation.[10] Later in gestation, the benefits of transfusion may be outweighed by the risks of delaying delivery. The transfusions are administered intravascularly. It is recommended to consider transfusion only when the fetal hematocrit falls below 30%.[10]

The transfused red cells are carefully selected to be type O, D-negative, and packed to achieve a hematocrit of 75–85%, thereby preventing volume overload. Additionally, the cells are irradiated to prevent any potential fetal graft-versus-host reactions and are purified to be leukocyte depleted to prevent cytomegalovirus infection.

The transfusion set consists of:

- Chiba needle (20 gauge)
- Blood transfusion set, three-way cannula, extension tubing, disposable sterile probe cover, 10 mL syringes, 5 mL syringes, and ethylenediaminetetraacetic acid (EDTA) vacutainers
- Injections xylocaine and vecuronium

- Normal saline, infusion set, and venflon **(Figs. 4A and B)**
- Maternal resuscitation set (intubation set, adrenaline, and atropine)

Before the transfusion procedure, a paralytic agent such as vecuronium/atracurium/pancuronium should be administered to the fetus as per the fetal weight to achieve quiescence. For nonhydropic fetuses, the target hematocrit typically ranges from 40 to 50%. The volume of blood to be transfused can be calculated by multiplying the estimated fetal weight in grams by 0.02 for each 10% increase required in hematocrit.[1]

The vascular access is preferred to be the cord insertion at placental site or intrahepatic portion of umbilical vein **(Figs. 5A and B)**. Initially, 1 mL of fetal blood is withdrawn to check the hematocrit and calculate the exact amount required to be transfused. Blood is transfused at a slow rate of 1 mL/min and a posttransfusion sample is obtained to check the final hematocrit achieved. After the transfusion is complete, fetal heart rate is checked for bradycardia and mother and fetus has to be monitored for 1 hour postprocedure.

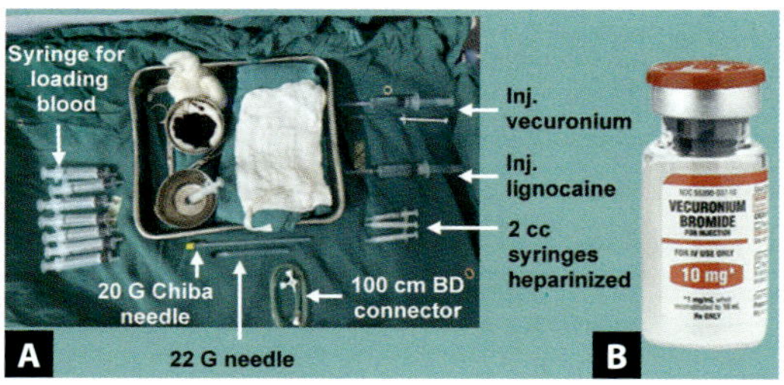

Figs. 4A and B: Intrauterine transfusion set with vecuronium (paralytic agent).

Fetal complications are bradycardia, cord hematoma (3–5%), fetal demise (2%), circulatory overload, and thromboembolism. Maternal complications can be preterm labor, premature rupture of membranes, chorioamnionitis, and formation of additional antibodies to newer antigens.

Follow-up: Post-IUT, the rate of fall of hematocrit is 1% per day after first IUT and reduces to 0.8–0.6% after consecutive procedures. The fetus is monitored to detect any signs of fetal anemia; MCA PSV sensitivity becomes low after multiple transfusions. The need for next IUT is decided based on the likely number of days in which fetal hematocrit will theoretically as per rate of fall reduce to 30%.

Outcome: The survival rate is estimated to be around 95%. If transfusion is necessary before the 20th week of gestation, the stillbirth rate surpasses 15%. In cases of hydropic fetuses, the neonatal survival rate is approximately 80%.[1]

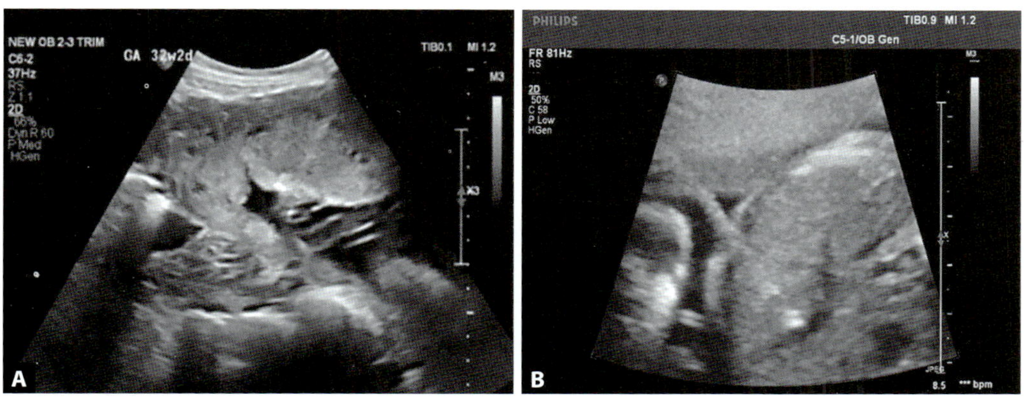

Figs. 5A and B: Procedure of intrauterine transfusion where the needle is seen: (A) In umbilical vein at placental cord insertion site; (B) In the umbilical vein in fetal liver.

Recent attention has been directed toward the utilization of maternal IVIG therapy to defer the requirement for initial IUT until after 20 weeks in pregnancies severely affected by anemia. Despite an unclear mechanism of action, IVIG therapy has demonstrated efficacy in postponing the necessity for transfusion by an average of 3 weeks and reducing the risk of hydrops.[1]

The management of Rh-negative pregnancy revolves around the proactive involvement of obstetricians in various facets. Obstetricians play a pivotal role in early detection through routine screening for Rh status during prenatal care, allowing timely intervention to prevent isoimmunization. Timely administration of anti-D immunoglobulin to Rh-negative women during pregnancy and postpartum mitigates the risk of isoimmunization following exposure to Rh-positive fetal blood. Obstetricians are the first contact of the pregnant mother and therefore, a close watch on the Rh-negative pregnancy for signs of isoimmunization is pivotal. Timely referral to a fetal medicine specialist should be done in order to provide appropriate interventions, such as IUT and manage fetal complications.

When to refer to a fetal medicine specialist?

- Women who have a previous history of pregnancies affected with severe neonatal jaundice/kernicterus, stillbirth
- Pregnancy with fetal anemia/hydrops
- Pregnancy with alloimmunization or positive antibody titers done with ICT
- Both Rh-negative couple with fetal or neonatal losses

Rhesus-negative women must be educated about the significance of anti-D prophylaxis, the risks associated with isoimmunization, and the importance of regular prenatal monitoring, ensures comprehensive care to optimize both maternal and fetal outcomes.

REFERENCES

1. Cunningham FG, Leveno KJ, Dashe JS, Hoffman BL, Spong CY, Casey BM (Eds). Williams Obstetrics, 26 edition. India: McGraw Hill; 2022.
2. RCOG. (2014). The Management of Women with Red Cell Antibodies during Pregnancy. Green-top Guideline No. 65. [online] Available from https://www.rcog.org.uk/media/oykp1rtg/rbc_gtg65.pdf [Last accessed April, 2024].
3. Mayekar RV, Paradkar GV, Bhosale AA, Sachan R, Beeram S, Anand AR, et al. Recombinant anti-D for prevention of maternal-foetal Rh(D) alloimmunization: a randomized multi-centre clinical trial. Obstet Gynecol Sci. 2020;63(3):315-22.
4. Practice Bulletin No. 181: Prevention of Rh D Alloimmunization. Obstet Gynecol. 2017;130(2):e57-e70.
5. FOGSI and TOG Conclave. Anti-D Immunoglobulin for Rh Prophylaxis: Key Practice Points. [online] Available from https://www.fogsi.org/wp-content/uploads/tog/anti-d-immunoglobulin-2022.pdf [Last accessed April, 2024].
6. Qureshi H, Massey E, Kirwan D, Davies T, Robson S, White J, et al. BCSH guideline for the use of anti-D immunoglobulin for the prevention of haemolytic disease of the fetus and newborn. Transfus Med. 2014;24(1):8-20.
7. World Health Organization. Abortion care guideline. Geneva: World Health Organization; 2022.
8. Visser GHA, Thommesen T, Di Renzo GC, Nassar AH, Spitalnik SL, Nassar A, et al. FIGO/ICM guidelines for preventing Rhesus disease: A call to action. Int J Gynecol Obstet. 2021;152(2):144-7.
9. Oepkes D, Seaward PG, Vandenbussche FP, Windrim R, Kingdom J, Beyene J, et al. Doppler ultrasonography versus amniocentesis to predict fetal anemia. N Engl J Med. 2006;355(2):156-64.
10. Mari G, Norton ME, Stone J, Berghella V, Sciscione AC, Tate D, et al. Society for Maternal-Fetal Medicine (SMFM) Clinical Guideline #8: The fetus at risk for anemia—diagnosis and management. Am J Obstet Gynecol. 2015;212(6):697-710.

13

CHAPTER

Nonimmune Hydrops Fetalis

Mounika Endrakanti, Neerja Gupta

KEY POINTS

1. Nonimmune hydrops fetalis (NIHF) is a pathological condition characterized by excessive collection of fluid in two or more fetal body compartments and affects about 1 in 2,000 pregnancies.
2. A diverse range of conditions that alter the fetal fluid dynamics are responsible for NIHF.
3. Detailed antenatal phenotyping and identification of unique and distinguishing manifestations in each case are invaluable in pinning down the etiology and thereby guide diagnostic testing.
4. Fetal exome sequencing is an important part of etiological evaluation, especially in cases undiagnosed by routine evaluation, with an approximate additional yield of about 29%.
5. Fetal autopsy is an integral part of NIHF workup, especially when next-generation sequencing is performed.
6. An algorithmic approach in the evaluation of these cases is recommended, as establishing a definite etiology is imperative for timely and effective management and anticipation of neonatal complications.
7. Multidisciplinary coordination and care are vital in pregnancies with NIHF in view of the significant morbidity and mortality associated with it.

INTRODUCTION

Fetal hydrops is a pathological condition characterized by excessive collection of fluid in fetal body compartments and interstitial tissues and, by definition, involves two or more serous cavities.[1] Traditionally, it is classified as immune hydrops and NIHF. NIHF affects about 1 in 2,000 pregnancies and is associated with high perinatal and neonatal morbidity and mortality.

DEFINITION

Fetal hydrops is generally detected by antenatal ultrasound and is defined as the presence of two or more abnormal fluid collections including pleural effusion, pericardial effusion, ascites, or generalized subcutaneous edema (thickness of the skin measuring >5 mm). The common associated ultrasonographic findings include polyhydramnios and thickening of the placenta (>4 or 6 cm in the second or third trimester, respectively).

PATHOPHYSIOLOGY

The underlying pathophysiology for fluid accumulation in NIHF includes an imbalance in the fluid dynamics between the interstitial fluid and vascular compartment, resulting from any or combination of the following four mechanisms **(Fig. 1)**:[2]

1. Increased capillary hydrostatic pressure
2. Reduced plasma oncotic pressure
3. Lymphatic flow obstruction
4. Altered integrity of peripheral capillaries

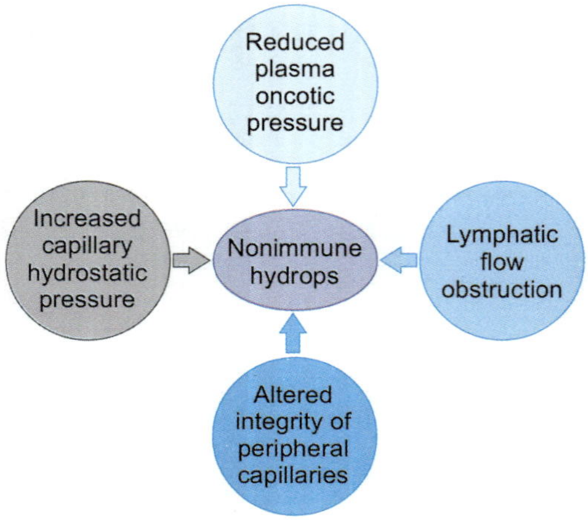

Fig. 1: Pathophysiology of fluid accumulation in nonimmune hydrops fetalis (NIHF).

ETIOLOGY

An etiology is usually identified in up to 60% of cases prenatally. The etiological spectrum of NIHF is diverse and includes a wide range of conditions as mentioned next and shown in **Figure 2**.

- *Cardiovascular abnormalities:* It is the most commonly reported etiology of NIHF (approximately 20%). These include structural heart diseases, fetal arrhythmias, cardiomyopathies, and vascular disorders.
  - *Structural heart diseases:* Right-sided defects are more commonly associated with hydrops owing to their direct effect on central venous pressure, as compared to left-sided lesions.
  - *Fetal arrhythmia:* Fetal tachyarrhythmias, most commonly supraventricular tachycardia, are associated with NIHF, resulting from increased central venous pressure and low cardiac output. Fetal bradycardia associated with congenital heart block secondary to transplacental passage of anti-Ro/SSA and anti-La/SSB antibodies in maternal autoimmune diseases such as systemic lupus erythematosus and Sjogren's syndrome may also present with hydrops.
  - *Cardiomyopathies*: Cardiomyopathies associated with lysosomal storage disorders (LSDs), Noonan syndrome, myocardial noncompaction, and endocardial fibroelastosis result in NIHF owing to myocardial dysfunction.
- *Genetic causes:* Genetic conditions contribute to a major proportion of NIHF and are associated with relatively poorer outcomes. These include the following:
  - *Chromosomal disorders:* A major proportion of NIHF detected in the first trimester result from chromosomal disorders (70%). Common aneuploidies like Turner syndrome and Down syndrome account for about 13% of the causes of NIHF, followed by trisomy 13, trisomy 18, and triploidy.
  - *Monogenic disorders:* The prevalence of monogenic disorders is higher during the second (20%) and third (20%) trimesters as compared to the first trimester (5%).[4] Monogenic conditions commonly associated with NIHF include inborn errors of metabolism, mainly LSDs and skeletal dysplasias. LSDs constitute up to 7–8% cases with NIHF. Common LSDs presenting with hydrops include mucopolysaccharidosis (MPS, commonly MPS VII), galactosialidosis, sialidosis, infantile-onset sialic acid storage disease, Gaucher disease, GM1 gangliosidosis, and Niemann–Pick disease.
- *Increased intrathoracic pressure:* Intrathoracic masses, lung malformations like congenital pulmonary airway malformation (CPAM), large fluid accumulations as in chylothorax, and hydrothorax lead to NIHF through impaired venous return.

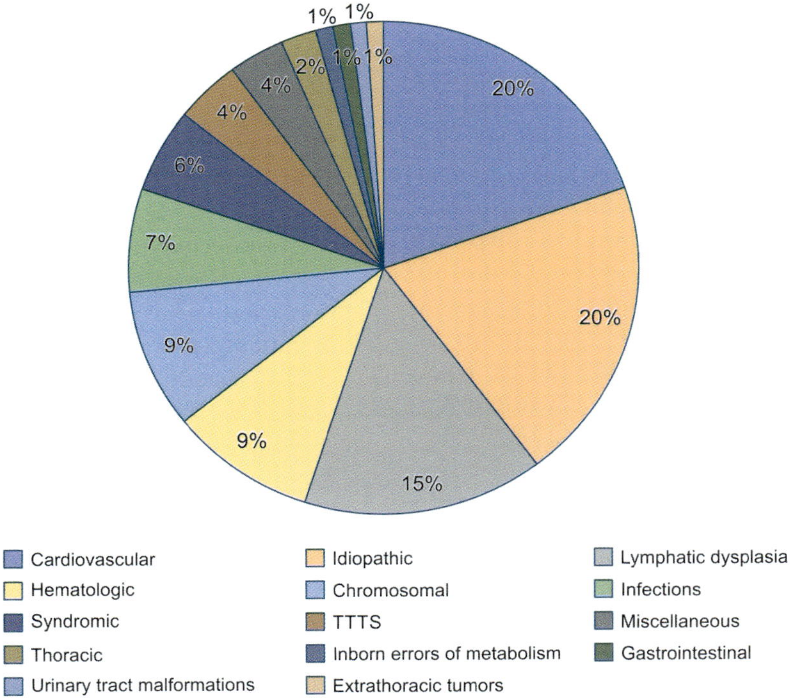

Fig. 2: Pie diagram depicting the etiological profile of NIHF. (NIHF: nonimmune hydrops fetalis; TTTS: twin-to-twin transfusion syndrome)
Source: Meta-analysis by Bellini et al.[2,3]

Chylothorax, a common cause of isolated effusion causing NIHF is often associated with a good prognosis for treatment.

- *Hematological conditions:* Hematological disorders characterized by destruction or loss of erythrocytes by hemolysis or hemorrhage or reduced production of erythrocytes may sometimes present with NIHF due to severe anemia and cardiac failure. These conditions include the following:
  - *Erythrocyte destruction or loss:* Hemolytic disorders due to hemoglobinopathies like homozygous α^0 thalassemia commonly, and rarely enzymopathies like glucose-6-phosphate dehydrogenase (G6PD) deficiency, glucose phosphate isomerase deficiency, and pyruvate kinase deficiency cause severe fetal anemia leading to NIHF. Homozygous α^0 thalassemia, an important hematological cause of NIHF, accounts for up to 50–80% of cases of NIHF and usually leads to fetal death in late gestation or the immediate postpartum period. Chronic fetomaternal hemorrhage, fetal hemangioma or arteriovenous malformations, fetal tumors like sacrococcygeal teratoma, and twin-to-twin transfusion syndrome (TTTS) are also associated with NIHF.
  - *Impaired erythrocyte production:* Bone marrow infiltration from conditions like transient myeloproliferative disorders, congenital leukemia, and bone marrow depression by intrauterine parvovirus B19 infection

are known to result in NIHF due to severe anemia. Parvovirus infection earlier than 20 weeks of gestation is associated with poorer outcomes and risk of abnormal neurodevelopmental outcomes despite transfusion.[5]

- *Infections:* Important clues on antenatal ultrasound in addition to hydrops, such as intrauterine growth retardation, ventriculomegaly, microcephaly, and hepatosplenomegaly may point to infectious causes of fetal hydrops. These mainly include parvovirus, cytomegalovirus, syphilis, toxoplasmosis, etc., accounting for 5–10% cases of NIHF. Congenital parvovirus B19 infection is associated with an increased risk of fetal loss, spontaneous abortion, and stillbirth, in the presence of hydrops as a presenting sign on ultrasound.[6]
- *Other systemic anomalies:* Structural renal and urinary anomalies including urethral obstruction, posterior urethral valve, renal agenesis and dysgenesis, congenital nephrosis, etc., are rare causes of fetal hydrops constituting up to 1% of cases. Gastrointestinal abnormalities constitute less common causes of NIHF (1.3%) and include intestinal stenosis, atresia, cirrhosis, etc. Abnormal development of lymphatics or lymphatic malformations like cystic hygroma resulting in impaired lymphatic drainage often occur as a component of chromosomal disorders. Heterotaxy syndromes associated with left atrial isomerism or complex congenital heart disease presenting with complete heart block causing early heart failure also present as fetal hydrops.
- *Inborn errors of immunity:* Fetal hydrops is the most common intrauterine manifestation noted in 70% cases of antenatally presenting familial hemophagocytic lymphohistiocytosis, a disorder characterized by functional deficit of cytotoxic T-cells and natural killer (NK) cells leading to immune dysregulation. Similarly, recurrent male fetal death with NIHF is a common presentation of IPEX syndrome, an X-linked condition characterized by immune dysregulation, polyendocrinopathy, and enteropathy. Hydrops is also an important antenatal manifestation of rare phagocyte dysfunction disorders like X-linked chronic granulomatous disease, complement deficiency disorders like 3MC syndrome, and interleukin-2 receptor β chain defect.[7]
- *TTTS*: Abnormal anastomoses within placental circulation leading to circulatory imbalance between twins result in TTTS. The presence of hydrops in TTTS is observed to result in a poor prognosis.
- The etiological spectrum of NIHF varies with gestation as shown in **Figure 3**. The onset of NIHF in the first trimester usually signifies a nonimmune etiology. Chromosomal abnormalities occur most commonly, constituting about 70% of cases presenting prior to 14 weeks of gestation. Onset of hydrops in the second trimester needs an urgent evaluation for fetal anemia as hematological causes are more common at this gestation. Cardiac structural anomalies (25%) and monogenic disorders (20%) are more common causes of hydrops in the third trimester.
- Idiopathic hydrops is four times more common in NIHF detected in the second and third trimesters as compared to the first trimester.[4]

APPROACH TO EVALUATION

A systematic multimodal prenatal and postnatal evaluation is essential in NIHF as an etiology is identified in up to 85%. The

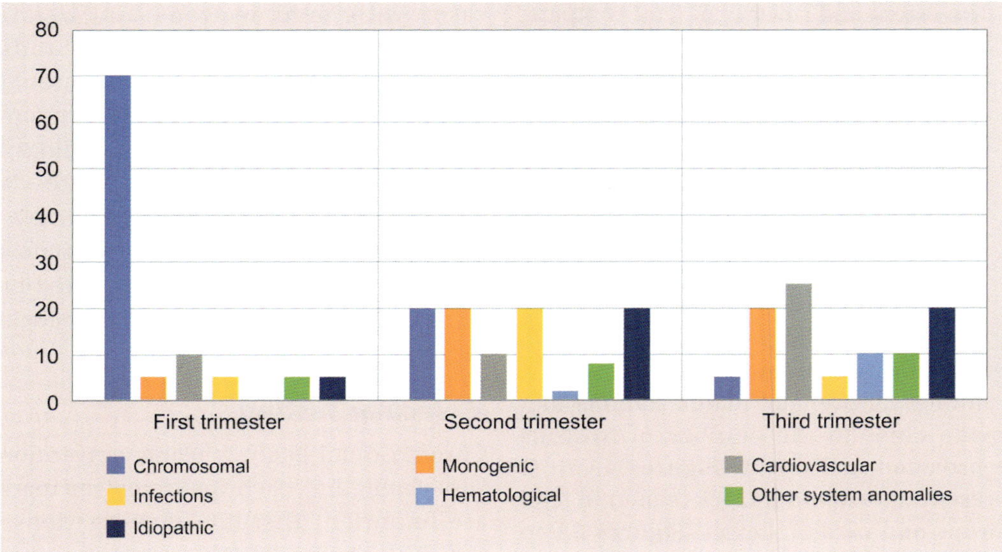

Fig. 3: Trimester-wise prevalence of various etiologies of nonimmune hydrops fetalis (NIHF) (percentage on *y*-axis).
Source: Modified from the review published by Khairudin et al. (2023).[4]

approach to the evaluation of fetal hydrops is as follows.

History and Maternal Evaluation

A detailed maternal medical, obstetric, and family history is the first step in evaluation. It is essential to enquire about the history of previous pregnancy losses/abortions, history of NIHF in a previous fetus/neonate, and obstetric evaluation/interventions performed if any. Family history concerning consanguinity, history of blood transfusions, proven genetic disorders, family members with developmental delay, early death, etc., may point toward a higher likelihood of genetic conditions. Enquiring about any recent illness, travel, contacts, and profession to assess the risk of recent infections that increase the risk of fetal hydrops like cytomegalovirus, parvovirus B19, and toxoplasmosis may also be useful.

Maternal evaluation includes monitoring for hypertension, abdominal discomfort, signs and symptoms of preeclampsia like edema and weight gain, and urine analysis for proteinuria. Maternal mirror syndrome is a maternal complication associated with fetal hydrops in the second and third trimesters, and also a close mimic to preeclampsia. It is characterized by maternal edema and placentomegaly (thickness >40 mm and >60 mm in second and third trimesters, respectively, placental edema). In addition to fetal hydrops, and is associated with high maternal morbidity and fetal mortality.[8] Screening for maternal hemoglobinopathies, especially alpha thalassemia (screen positive if mean cell volume of the parents <80 fL), and viral infections such as toxoplasma, cytomegalovirus, and parvovirus B19 is also indicated.

Radiological Evaluation

Detailed antenatal fetal evaluation by 2D and 3D ultrasonogram is important to assess and monitor:

- The extent and severity of fetal compartments involved
- Structural anomalies including skeletal abnormalities
- Fetal growth and well-being
- Signs of fetal anemia (elevated middle cerebral artery peak systolic velocity >1.5 MoM in second and third trimesters)
- Placental thickness and appearance
- Adequacy of liquor
- Fetal echocardiogram to evaluate for structural cardiac anomalies

Additional prenatal manifestations that provide clues to the etiology of hydrops are provided in **Table 1**. **Figures 4A to D** represent ultrasound images related to fetal hydrops and cardiac defect. **Figures 5A to D** show the representative images of fetuses with NIHF due to chromosomal and single-gene disorders.

Fetal Blood Sampling

Fetal blood sampling is especially useful in cases with fetal anemia. Alpha thalassemia is an important cause of anemia in fetuses with NIHF presenting in the second or third trimester, and accounts for 28–55% of the cases of NIHF in Southeast Asian population.[1]

Evaluation of Body Fluids

Evaluation of pleural fluid/ascitic fluid is sometimes useful for etiological evaluation. The important pointers include:

- Lymphocyte predominance (>80%) in chylous effusions[1]
- Vacuolated lymphocytes in glycogen storage disorders
- Low protein in urinary ascites
- Elevated gamma-glutamyl transferase (GGT) in bowel perforation.

Fetal Autopsy

Although an initial diagnosis of NIHF is usually made on an antenatal ultrasonogram, cases with mild hydrops and delayed onset may often be missed. Studies report discrepancies between antenatal ultrasonogram and fetal or neonatal autopsy, with the detection of additional findings on autopsy in approximately 35% of cases. It is therefore preferable to perform an autopsy in all cases of NIHF resulting in fetal or neonatal loss, as any additional findings noted may result in a higher diagnostic yield and redefine the recurrence risk.[9,10]

Molecular Testing

Chromosomal analysis using conventional karyotyping and/or chromosomal microarray are important first-line investigations in the evaluation of NIHF as chromosomal abnormalities are the most common genetic causes accounting for 27–38%.[9,11,12]

The overall diagnostic yield of whole exome sequencing (WES) in NIHF is about 37%.[13] In cases with unexplained NIHF, fetal WES has an additional diagnostic yield of about 29%. The presence of additional features is observed to result in higher yield as compared to isolated NIHF.[9,10] A similar incremental diagnostic yield (23%) has been reported from trio clinical ES in NIHF cases with inconclusive routine etiological work-up.[14] Among monogenic conditions associated with hydrops, RASopathies (24–30%) and neuromuscular disorders (21%), metabolic (17%), and musculoskeletal conditions (14.5%) are the most common.[10,13] The yield of WES is not observed to correspond to the severity of hydrops or family history (recurrent vs. simplex cases). Although autosomal dominant conditions resulting from *de novo* monoallelic pathogenic variants are more common in simplex cases of NIHF, autosomal recessive disorders are common in predominantly consanguineous cohorts and multiplex families.[9,10]

TABLE 1: Additional prenatal manifestations that provide clues to the etiology of nonimmune hydrops fetalis (NIHF).

Additional prenatal manifestations (in addition to NIHF)	***Likely etiology***
Fetal anemia	• Alpha thalassemia (HbH and Hb Barts) • Congenital dyserythropoietic anemia • G6PD deficiency • Glucose phosphate isomerase deficiency • Pyruvate kinase deficiency
Cystic hygroma	• Turner syndrome (monosomy X) (often septated) • Edwards syndrome (trisomy 18) • Noonan syndrome • Lethal multiple pterygium syndrome • Congenital erythropoietic porphyria • Generalized lymphatic dysplasia
Chylothorax	• Noonan syndrome • Yellow nail syndrome • ITGA9-associated fetal chylothorax
Cardiac anomalies: • Endocardial cushion defects • Coarctation of aorta • Hypertrophic cardiomyopathy • Dilated cardiomyopathy	 • Down syndrome • Turner syndrome • Noonan syndrome, CDG type 1 • Barth syndrome
Fetal hepatosplenomegaly	Lysosomal storage disorders
Duodenal atresia	Down syndrome
Echogenic kidneys	• Autosomal recessive polycystic kidney disease • Congenital erythropoietic porphyria • IPEX syndrome
Hypoplastic cerebellum	• CDG • Congenital erythropoietic porphyria
Bowed long bones, beaded ribs	Osteogenesis imperfecta
Short ribs, narrow thorax, and polydactyly	Short rib polydactyly syndromes (types I–IV)
Fetal akinesia	• Pena–Shokier syndrome • Lethal multiple pterygium syndrome • Myotonic dystrophy • Neu–Laxova syndrome
Placentomegaly	• Congenital nephrotic syndrome (Finnish type) • Alpha thalassemia (HbH and Hb Barts) • MPS VII, Niemann Pick C disease (rare) • Lymphedema–cholestasis syndrome (Aagenaes syndrome) (rare)
Isolated hydrops	MPS IVA
Dark brown amniotic fluid	Congenital erythropoietic porphyria

(CDG: congenital disorders of glycosylation; G6PD: glucose-6-phosphate dehydrogenase; HbH: hemoglobin H; IPEX: immune dysregulation, polyendocrinopathy, enteropathy, X-linked; ITGA9: integrin alpha 9; MPS: mucopolysaccharidosis)

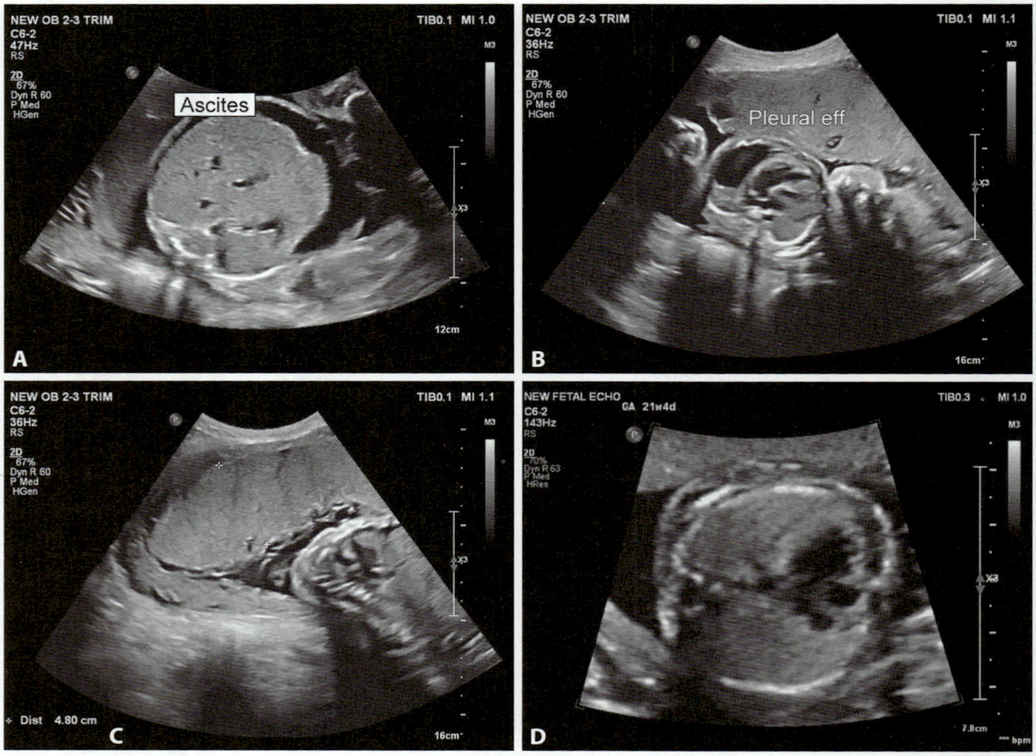

Figs. 4A to D: (A) Fetal ascites; (B) Fetal pleural effusion; (C) Placentomegaly; (D) Fetal cardiac atrioventricular septal defect.

An algorithmic approach to NIHF is depicted in **Flowchart 1**.

MANAGEMENT

Multidisciplinary coordination and care are vital in pregnancies with NIHF in view of the significant fetal morbidity and mortality associated with it. Prematurity and polyhydramnios are common in pregnancies with fetal hydrops, with an incidence of about 29% and 66% respectively.

As fetal therapies in potentially treatable conditions help improve perinatal outcomes, a prompt referral to tertiary care centers well equipped in fetal or early neonatal interventions is vital. A careful expectant management is indicated in cases with an anticipated favorable perinatal outcome, idiopathic hydrops, and those amenable to postnatal therapies. It is important to take precautions to ensure optimal fetal viability and survival, especially in pregnancies with progressive NIHF. Preterm delivery is recommended in NIHF only for obstetric indications. In pregnancies with nonprogressive NIHF, a term delivery around 37–38 weeks' gestation is advisable. Immediate delivery may be necessitated in those with mirror syndrome. Various fetal therapies are shown in **Table 2**.

PROGNOSIS AND OUTCOMES

Most fetuses with hydrops succumb before reaching viability, with mortality ranging

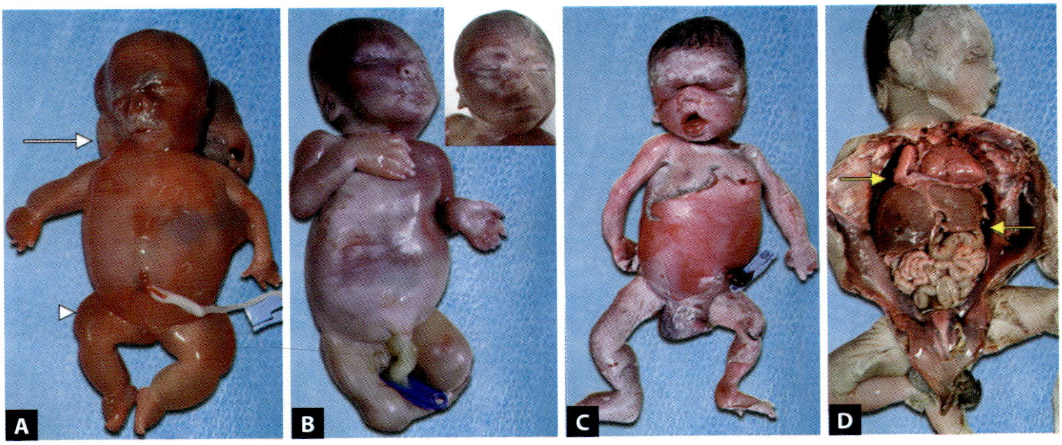

Figs. 5A to D: Representative images showing fetuses with chromosomal and single-gene disorders presenting with nonimmune hydrops. (A) A 19-week fetus with abnormal level II ultrasonogram showing fetal hydrops and cystic hygroma (white arrow) and generalized subcutaneous edema (white arrowhead). Prenatal testing by amniocentesis and karyotyping on cultured amniocytes suggested Turner syndrome (45,X0); (B) A 19-week fetus with antenatal findings of echogenic kidneys and hydronephrosis, and postnatal evaluation suggestive of hydrops, facial dysmorphism including flat facial profile, upslanted palpebral fissures, depressed nose and long philtrum, pleural effusion, and pericardial effusion. Testing by amniocentesis and karyotyping on cultured amniocytes suggested Down syndrome (trisomy 21); (C and D) Fetus with hydrops detected at 30 weeks of gestation and intrauterine demise at 35 weeks, and postnatal evaluation showing macerated fetus with pleural effusion and ascites (yellow arrows). Molecular testing by exome sequencing showed a hemizygous variant c.281G>A (p.Arg94His) in *TAZ*, causative of Barth syndrome.

between 35 and 98%. Gestational age at detection of NIHF and etiology play an important role in prognosis and survival with a greater risk in those detected at an earlier gestation. NIHF confers a mortality risk of up to 60% among liveborn infants with NIHF, with prematurity and significant illness immediately after birth posing the highest risk. Etiology wise, treatable causes like fetal cardiac conduction abnormalities and parvovirus B19 infection have better prognosis. Chromosomal abnormalities, genetic disorders, and inborn errors of metabolism presenting with NIHF have poor prognosis with high mortality. Survival in cardiovascular abnormalities often depends on the type of defect, with higher mortality in vascular disorders. Other important independent risk factors influencing the mortality in a neonate with NIHF include delivery at <34 weeks of gestational age, hypoalbuminemia (<2 g/dL), severe acidosis, lower APGAR score at 5 minutes, and requirement of high-frequency ventilation or high-level oxygen support on the first day of life. Response to fetal therapy (medical, percutaneous, or fetoscopic) and resolution of hydrops are important predictors of survival.

COUNSELING

Genetic counseling is an integral part of the management of pregnancies with NIHF. Counseling of these couples should follow an individualized approach focused on providing information about the prognosis,

Flowchart 1: Algorithmic approach to NIHF.

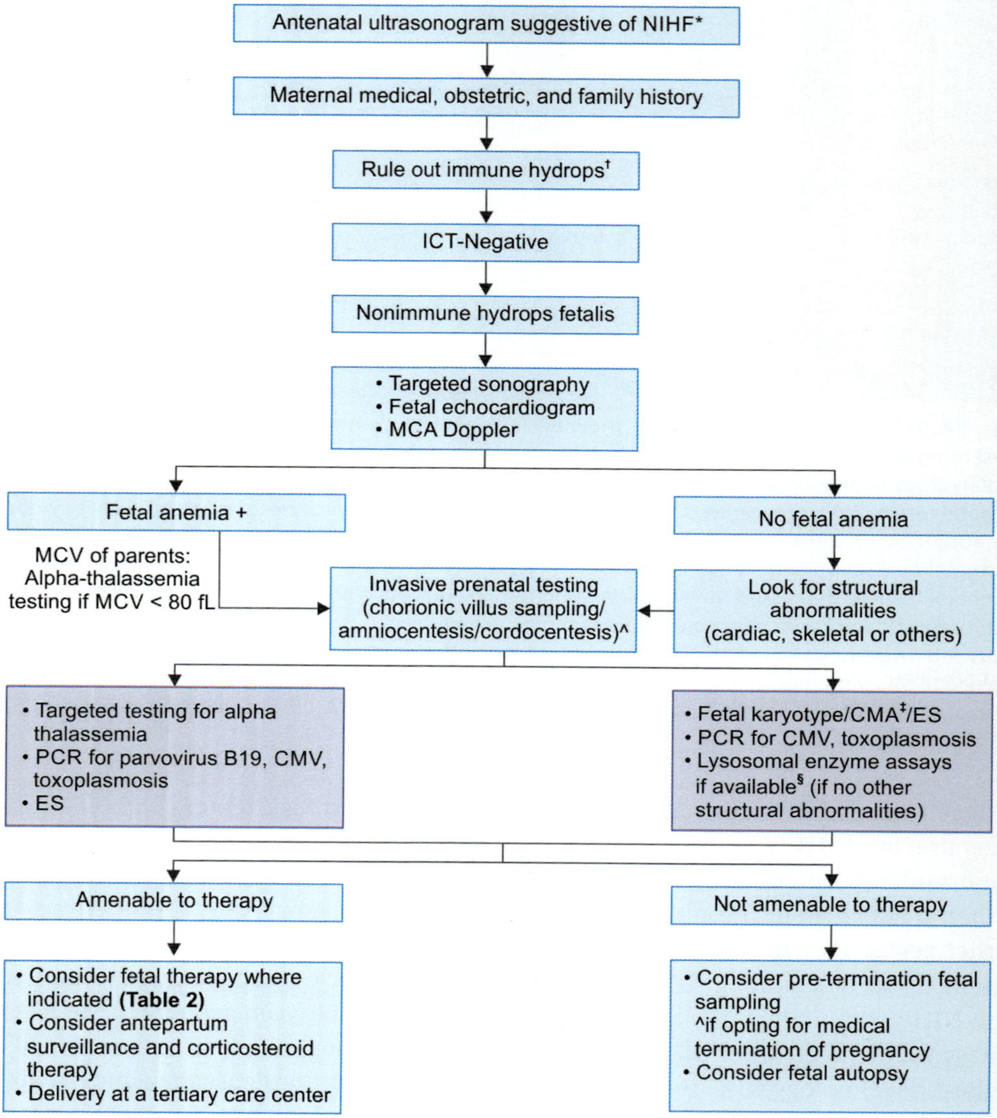

*Defined as the presence of two or more abnormal fluid collections.

†Using indirect Coombs test.

‡Regardless of the presence or absence of a fetal structural anomaly.

§Enzyme assays for common lysosomal storage disorders presenting with NIHF including mucopolysaccharidosis type VII, Gaucher disease, and GM1 gangliosidosis.

(CMA: chromosomal microarray; CMV: cytomegalovirus; ES: exome sequencing; ICT: indirect Coombs test; MCA: middle cerebral artery; MCV: mean corpuscular volume; NIHF: nonimmune hydrops fetalis; PCR: polymerase chain reaction)

Source: SMFM Clinical Guidelines for Nonimmune Hydrops Fetalis.[1]

TABLE 2: Fetal therapies in various causes of NIHF.

Condition	***Recommendation of fetal therapy***
Fetal anemia: • Fetomaternal hemorrhage • Parvovirus infection	Intrauterine transfusion following fetal blood sampling
Cardiac arrhythmia: • Supraventricular tachycardia • Atrial fibrillation • Atrial flutter	Maternal administration of antiarrhythmic agents is indicated unless gestation is advanced or maternal contraindication to antiarrhythmic agents exists
Critical aortic stenosis evolving to hypoplastic left heart syndrome	Fetal aortic valvuloplasty
Pulmonary atresia with intact ventricular septum	Fetal pulmonary valvuloplasty
CPAM	• *Microcystic CPAM:* Maternal administration of corticosteroids dexamethasone 4 mg per oral daily for 6 days or 6 mg intramuscular every 12 hours for 2 days, total dose being 24 mg • *Macrocystic CPAM:* Needle drainage of effusion or thoracoamniotic shunt placement
Fetal hydrothorax Fetal chylothorax Large pleural effusion associated with pulmonary sequestration	• Needle drainage of effusion (thoracocentesis) may be performed prior to delivery in those with large effusion • Thoracoamniotic shunt placement indicated in pleural effusion due to fetal lung lesion, rapid reaccumulation of pleural effusion, progressive polyhydramnios
Megacystic with normal renal function (normal urinary electrolyte profile)	• Vesicoamniotic shunt • Fetal cystoscopy
TTTS	Fetoscopic laser ablation of anastomosis in the placenta is indicated in NIHF associated with TTTS prior to 26 weeks' gestation
TRAP	Percutaneous radiofrequency ablation
Tumors: • Placental chorioangioma • Head and neck mass	• In utero surgical resection/radiofrequency ablation • EXIT procedure

(CPAM: congenital pulmonary airway malformation; EXIT: ex utero intrapartum treatment; NIHF: nonimmune hydrops fetalis; TRAP: twin-reversed arterial perfusion; TTTS: twin-to-twin transfusion syndrome)

potential risks, and outcomes based on the etiology, its severity, and timing of detection, especially for those with potentially treatable conditions. Comprehensive evaluation including molecular diagnosis should be offered for all couples. Establishing a genetic diagnosis antenatally may prove vital in guiding the course of pregnancy. It is also helpful to the couple in the decision-making process, understanding the risk of recurrence and reproductive options for future pregnancies.

REFERENCES

1. Norton ME, Chauhan SP, Dashe JS. Society for Maternal-Fetal Medicine (SMFM) Clinical Guideline #7: nonimmune hydrops fetalis. Am J Obstet Gynecol. 2015;212(2):127-39.
2. Swearingen C, Colvin ZA, Leuthner SR. Nonimmune Hydrops Fetalis. Clin Perinatol. 2020;47(1):105-21.
3. Bellini C, Donarini G, Paladini D, Calevo MG, Bellini T, Ramenghi LA, et al. Etiology of non-immune hydrops fetalis: An update. Am J Med Genet A. 2015;167A(5):1082-8.
4. Khairudin D, Alfirevic Z, Mone F, Navaratnam K. Non-immune hydrops fetalis: a practical guide for obstetricians. Obstet Gynaecol. 2023;25(2):110-20.
5. Nagel HTC, de Haan TR, Vandenbussche FPHA, Oepkes D, Walther FJ. Long-term outcome after fetal transfusion for hydrops associated with parvovirus B19 infection. Obstet Gynecol. 2007;109(1):42-7.
6. Xiong YQ, Tan J, Liu YM, He Q, Li L, Zou K, et al. The risk of maternal parvovirus B19 infection during pregnancy on fetal loss and fetal hydrops: A systematic review and meta-analysis. J Clin Virol. 2019;114:12-20.
7. Carneiro-Sampaio M, de Jesus AA, Bando SY, Moreira-Filho CA. Inborn errors of immunity with fetal or perinatal clinical manifestations. Front Pediatr. 2022;10:891343.
8. Han Z, Chen X, Wang Q, Zhou J, Guo Y, Hou H, et al. Clinical characteristics and risk factors of mirror syndrome: a retrospective case-control study. BMC Pregnancy Childbirth. 2021;21(1):660.
9. Correa ARE, Naini K, Mishra P, Dadhwal V, Agarwal R, Shukla R, et al. Utility of fetal whole exome sequencing in the etiological evaluation and outcome of nonimmune hydrops fetalis. Prenat Diagn. 2021;41(11):1414-24.
10. Mone F, Eberhardt RY, Hurles ME, Mcmullan DJ, Maher ER, Lord J, et al. Fetal hydrops and the Incremental yield of Next-generation sequencing over standard prenatal Diagnostic testing (FIND) study: prospective cohort study and meta-analysis. Ultrasound Obstet Gynecol. 2021;58(4):509-18.
11. Sparks TN, Thao K, Lianoglou BR, Boe NM, Bruce KG, Datkhaeva I, et al. Nonimmune hydrops fetalis: identifying the underlying genetic etiology. Genet Med. 2019;21(6):1339-44.
12. Laterre M, Bernard P, Vikkula M, Sznajer Y. Improved diagnosis in nonimmune hydrops fetalis using a standardized algorithm. Prenatal Diag. 2018;38(5):337-43.
13. Al-Kouatly HB, Shivashankar K, Mossayebi MH, Makhamreh M, Critchlow E, Gao Z, et al. Diagnostic yield from prenatal exome sequencing for non-immune hydrops fetalis: A systematic review and meta-analysis. Clin Genet. 2023;103(5):503-12.
14. Al-Kouatly HB, Makhamreh MM, Rice SM, Smith K, Harman C, Quinn A, et al. High diagnosis rate for nonimmune hydrops fetalis with prenatal clinical exome from the Hydrops-Yielding Diagnostic Results of Prenatal Sequencing (HYDROPS) Study. Genetics in Medicine. 2021;23(7):1325-33.

CHAPTER 14

Fetal Diagnostic Procedures

Reema Bhatt, Veronica Arora

KEY POINTS

1. Invasive prenatal techniques play a crucial role in determining whether a fetus is normal.
2. Amniocentesis, chorionic villus sampling (CVS), and cordocentesis can now be performed within the parameters of accepted practices, which include complications, checklists, suggested procedures, local legal requirements, counseling, and clear and reliable indications.
3. These procedures should be performed at specified period of gestation to optimize the results and reduce complications.
4. These procedures can also be performed with proper equipment and training.
5. There has been a significant drop in the probability of fetal loss after invasive prenatal diagnostic testing.
6. Quality control shall be ensured by appropriate training, adherence to this document's standards, and periodical audit processes.

INTRODUCTION

Prenatal invasive diagnostic testing is an essential and incredibly important part of providing optimal care of fetus. We need to provide pregnant women and their family with management options making educated informed decisions to determine the health of fetus.

With the right training and tools, amniocentesis, CVS, and cordocentesis can now be carried out within the bounds of accepted practices, which include clear and reliable indications, counseling, informed consents, local legal requirements, checklists, suggested procedures, and complications. Following prenatal diagnostic invasive testing, the likelihood of fetal loss has considerably decreased in recent years.

We will consider three important diagnostic procedures: (1) Amniocentesis, (2) CVS, and (3) cordocentesis.

REASONS OF PRENATAL TESTING

The following are the typical justifications for undergoing invasive prenatal tests:

- A positive prenatal aneuploidy screening result such as maternal serum analytes with or without sonographic aneuploidy markers or cell-free deoxyribonucleic acid (DNA)
- Pronounced nuchal translucency
- Congenital abnormality discovered via ultrasonography
- A sex chromosome related sickness is carried by the female parent.
- Either parent is a carrier of an autosomal dominant or recessive monogenic (also known as single gene or Mendelian) condition.
- Both parents carry a gene known to cause a genetic illness.

A balanced translocation or another structural chromosomal abnormality is carried by the parent.

- A previous child who had a diagnosed intellectual handicap, metabolic condition, congenital defect, or chromosome abnormalities
- Mothers who were 35 years or older at the anticipated due date
- Hemoglobinopathies
- Disorders related to sex

There are certain preprocedure prerequisites that need to be adhered to:

History:

- Age, infectious diseases, obstetric history, family history of genetic diseases, chronic medical disorders, and medication history should be elicited in detail.[1]
- Where applicable, specifics on in vitro fertilization (IVF), ovum donation, the age of the ovum donor, and surrogacy should be mentioned.

It is important to determine the mother's Rhesus (Rh) status. Counseling for the administration of prophylactic anti-D immunoglobulin within 72 hours of the procedure if the patient is Rh negative unless the father of the fetus is known to be Rh negative.[2]

A woman with human immunodeficiency virus (HIV) who is on antiretroviral therapy (ART) and has a low/undetectable viral load significantly lowers her risk of vertical transmission. Prior to the procedure at least 2 weeks of ART are preferred.[3]

As far as thromboprophylaxis is concerned, there are not enough facts to stop giving thromboprophylaxis before invasive procedures on fetuses; however, a single dose of therapeutic heparin may be skipped.[4,5] There have been two schools of thought about the use of antibiotic. In a single randomized controlled trial (RCT), azithromycin was found to improve outcomes; however, the study's methodology had a number of flaws.[6] A smaller retrospective analysis found no difference in antibiotic use.[7]

Preprocedure planning of site by ultrasound is essential for the purposes of finding the placenta, determining gestational age, determining the amount of amniotic fluid present, and recording fetal heart rate.[8]

Pretest counseling should be in detail whenever an invasive procedure is planned.

This includes a description of the procedure's indications in a language that the patient and their partner can comprehend and acknowledge. The indication needs to fit into one of the forms F categories. Verbal descriptions or illustrations of the intended course of action, including any complications. The patient's need for and choice of the level of genetic testing analysis **(Table 1)**: The need for a second tier of genetic testing must be communicated, for instance, the requirement for exome sequencing if the microarray is clear. Information on the detection rates and restrictions of the specific laboratory test(s) being performed, the likelihood of inconclusive results and test failure rates, and the amount of time the laboratory needs to conduct the test(s) and provide the results. Option and a strategy for dealing with unfavorable test findings. Patients should be made expressly aware of whether the laboratory work-up is done internally or outside. The requirement to consult a doctor when test findings are made public, as well as management alternatives after the results. The requirement for postprocedure anti-D passive immunization if the lady is Rh negative and unvaccinated. Following this thorough informational procedure, the woman should sign written consent forms under the testimony of a signatory. It is necessary to get both Form G and the general consent form.

TABLE 1: Tests conducted on prenatal samples.

Sr. no.	Tests for	TAT	Resolution	Advantages	Limitations
1. Karyotype	• Chromosomal abnormalities • Missing/extra chromosomal material, ring chromosomes, isochromosomes, markers, and mosaicism	3 weeks	>5.5 MB	• Gold standard • Test for aneuploidies, polyploidies • Affordable, characterizes abnormalities like marker or ring chromosome	• Miss microdeletion, microduplications • Low level mosaicism, does not pick up maternal cell contamination
2. FISH	Targeted areas of genomes	2 days	0.5 MB	Quick results	• Expensive • Needs targeted probes, cannot screen all regions together, does not pick up maternal cell contamination
3. QFPCR	Aneuploidies, MCC	2–5 days	–	Quick	Picks maternal cell contamination, type of aneuploidy
4. CMA	Chromosomal abnormalities	10 days	20 kb Copy number variations	Picks up small deletions or duplications	Array CGH misses triploidy, does not tell the type of Down syndrome, misses balanced translocations
5. Exome	Monogenic disorders (only the protein coding region)	3–6 weeks	1 bp	Picks up inversions, SNPs, small deletions, mosaicism	Misses larger deletions, presence of VOUS

(CGH: comparative genomic hybridization; CMA: chromosomal microarray analysis; FISH: fluorescence in situ hybridization; MCC: maternal cell contamination; QFPCR: quantitative fluorescent polymerase chain reaction; SNPs: single nucleotide polymorphisms; TAT: turnaround time; VOUS: variants of uncertain significance)

PROCEDURE DETAILS

Chorionic Villus Sampling

Small samples of the placenta are taken through a process called CVS in order to do prenatal genetic diagnostics. It is a safe and efficient procedure when used by qualified personnel. It is often carried out after 10 weeks gestation in the first trimester. Early CVS is not advised due to a higher risk of pregnancy loss and problems with limb reduction.[4,9,10] Either the transcervical (TC) technique or the percutaneous transabdominal (TA) approach can be used to execute it.

The CVS has benefits over amniocentesis, considering that villi can typically be directly subjected to biochemical or DNA analysis, negating the need for cell culture which is necessary following amniocentesis. Secondly, the CVS sample produces substantially more DNA than 20 mL of amniotic fluid and CVS causes a move toward early diagnosis, giving the couple precious time to make decisions.

Technique

The patient is positioned supine and has her lower abdomen cleaned with an antiseptic solution before undergoing TA-CVS. The TA-CVS procedure is accompanied by a little discomfort. No data exists to demonstrate that analgesia before CVS lessens pain. Since its use only produces cutaneous anesthesia and not uterine wall penetration anesthesia, such studies did not demonstrate any pain reduction by prior administration of analgesia or local anesthesia. In general, women undergoing amniocentesis could be told that the procedure causes very mild discomfort, and the Cochrane review found that there is currently insufficient data to warrant the use of local anesthesia.[11] "Pain scores" were lower in the analgesia group in one randomized control experiment, albeit this difference did not achieve statistical significance. For CVS, the same would be true.

The needle size that is utilized (18-gauge, 20-gauge, double-needle 17/19-gauge, double-needle 18/21-gauge), as well as the aspiration technique (negative pressure by syringe, negative pressure by vacuum aspirator, biopsy forceps), differs significantly among TA-CVS techniques.

Either a free-hand approach or a needle-guide connected to the ultrasonic probe is used to place the needle. The author favors the use of a freehand method and an 18-gauge spinal needle **(Fig. 1)**. The placenta's long axis can be penetrated by the needle because it is advanced at an angle **(Figs. 2A and B)**. The stylet is taken out, the 20-cc syringe containing the medium is positioned on the holder, and finally the holder is fastened to the needle's hub. Up until a sufficient sample is sucked by

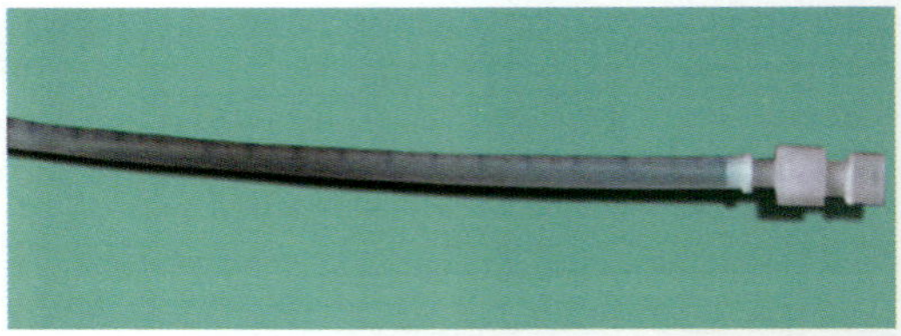

Fig. 1: 18-gauge spinal needle.

the syringe's vacuum, the needle tip is pushed back and forth inside the placenta **(Fig. 2C)**. Next, the sample apparatus is removed while being compressed downward **(Fig. 2D)**.

Transcervical CVS is becoming less common due to its technical difficulty, according to a recent survey.[12]

The amount of villi that was obtained is evaluated visually for sufficiency. For a microarray or karyotyping, 5–10 mg of villi is typically sufficient.[13]

Amniocentesis

Amniocentesis is conducted most effectively after 16 weeks of gestation. Early amniocentesis is a procedure that should be avoided since it has a higher risk of fetal loss and complications, such as culture failure and increased tenting of membranes.[14] In some situations, such as when fetal abnormalities are found late in gestation, late second- and third-trimester procedures for genetic studies are carried out because the knowledge can be helpful for counseling and preparing parents, as well as for planning the ideal time, route, and site of delivery.

Technique

Aseptic measures are followed during the process. Transabdominally, a 9-cm long, 22-gauge needle is inserted into an amniotic fluid pocket that is free of any parts of the fetus **(Fig. 3)** and the umbilical cord under real-time ultrasound monitoring by freehand technique.[4]

route, maintaining the fetoplacental circulation, following which the uterine incision is closed and the pregnancy is allowed to continue until term. It is indicated in cases of fetal lung masses (isolated CPAM—predominantly solid or multicystic) with hydrops which can have close to 100% fatality, fetal sacrococcygeal teratoma complicated by progressive high-output cardiac failure and <32 weeks' gestation when the tumor is anatomically amenable to resection. The potential postoperative complications specific to open fetal surgery include PPROM, chorioamniotic separation, and preterm labor.

SUGGESTED READING

1. Evans LL, Harrison MR. Modern fetal surgery—a historical review of the happenings that shaped modern fetal surgery and its practices. Transl Pediatr. 2021;10(5): 1401-17.
2. Harrison MR, Adzick NS. The fetus as a patient. Surgical considerations. Am Surg. 1991;213(4):279-91; discussion 277-8.
3. Maselli KM, Badillo A. Advances in fetal Surgery. Ann Transl Med. 2016;4(20):394.
4. Moreira de Sá RA, Nassar de Carvalho PR, Kurjak A, Adra A, Dayyabu AL, Ebrashy A, et al. Is intrauterine surgery justified? Report from the working group on ultrasound in obstetrics of the World Association of Perinatal Medicine (WAPM). J Perinat Med. 2016;44(7):737-43.
5. Sampat K, Losty PD. Fetal Surgery. Brit J Surg. 2021;108(6):632-7.

16

CHAPTER

Stillbirth and Fetal Autopsy

Sunil Jaiman

KEY POINTS

1. A combination of different factors lead to a stillbirth.
2. Fetal autopsy, placental pathology, and genetic testing are the most useful diagnostic tests following a stillbirth.
3. These investigations following a stillbirth are tailored to the clinical scenario, and a synergistic multidisciplinary collaboration of different specialists (obstetricians, neonatologists, pathologists, and geneticists) improves their detection.
4. The cause of stillbirth identification greatly facilitates emotional healing and provides closure for families.
5. The cause of stillbirth identification provides recurrence risk and future pregnancy management information to the healthcare providers and is most helpful in counseling the families.

INTRODUCTION

Stillbirth is often unpredictable and an agonizing adverse obstetric outcome, devastating for both the mother (parents) and the healthcare provider. The fetus is not accessible to most diagnostic tools and therefore, postmortem and placental examination in the case of stillbirth are most crucial as these investigations will most likely yield a cause of death.

Perinatal pathology, which encompasses fetal and perinatal autopsy and placental pathology, remains an invaluable tool in the evaluation of stillbirths (fetal deaths that occur after 20 weeks of gestation). The biggest challenge of perinatal pathology, however, is in acquiring maximal diagnostic information, when there is minimal knowledge of preceding events leading to stillbirth, the so-called unexplained stillbirth. The difficulties are further compounded when there is a delay between fetal death and delivery. Most often, the information regarding the timing of death is limited. Distinguishing between pathological changes which precede a stillbirth and autolytic changes, which follow a stillbirth are difficult. Moreover, following a stillbirth, the maceration process obscures tissue structural details.

Despite the challenges, a meticulous perinatal fetal autopsy and placental examination remains the most important diagnostic tool employed by healthcare providers. In this chapter, we will briefly discuss the role of fetal autopsy in stillbirth.

PERINATAL AUTOPSY

What are the Benefits of a Perinatal Autopsy?

The benefits of perinatal autopsy include: (1) Establishing the cause of stillbirth; (2) helping with bereavement closure; (3) documenting fetal growth and development; (4) providing future pregnancy stillbirth risk estimates; (5) unmasking of underlying pregnancy-related conditions; (6) corroborating or supplementing or refuting a clinical diagnosis; (7) identifying rare disease entities; (8) discovering newer pathologic entities;

(9) documenting previously unknown information on disease manifestations; (10) understanding of the genetic factors contributing to the stillbirth; (11) identifying infections or infectious etiology in a stillbirth; (12) contributing to research and education; (13) providing epidemiological data that can help understand the factors influencing perinatal mortality rates and thereby improving prenatal care; (14) improving healthcare practices such as prenatal screening methods and management of high-risk pregnancies, thereby potentially reducing the incidence of stillbirths in the future; (15) facilitating the investigation of environmental, occupational, and lifestyle causes of stillbirth; and (16) assessing the placental pathology to provide insight into placental insufficiency, infection, or other abnormalities that may have contributed to the stillbirth.

Perinatal autopsies are performed with the consent of the parents and the process is conducted with sensitivity and respect for the grieving family. Cultural, religious, or personal beliefs may influence the parents; therefore, the decision to perform an autopsy should be discussed and agreed upon with the family in a compassionate and understanding manner.

What is Informed Consent and Turnaround Time?

Obtaining an informed consent is the first single most important step in stillbirth evaluation. The patient may consent for either a complete fetal and placental evaluation without limitations or provide a partial consent that may include specified restrictions to the procedure. It may be pertinent to mention that most hospitals may have different consent forms for stillbirth evaluation, with varying requirements for additional procedures such as removal of the brain and spinal cord. The disposition of the fetus and the placenta upon the completion of the postmortem examination is determined by the patient or the family.

General turnaround time for a provisional and a final report is determined by the pathologist.

External and internal gross examination findings may be completed within 2–3 working days of receipt of the fetus and the placenta. The microscopic examination may be completed within 30 days.

The pathologists are provided with the informed consents and all other relevant and available clinical information along with the fetus and the placenta. If not provided, the prosector pathologist must actively seek all relevant clinical and family history prior to the procedure. The clinical and preautopsy considerations include obtaining a complete obstetric history, ultrasound reports, including those pertaining to prior pregnancies, and information about known genetic syndromes within the family.

Radiographic Imaging

X-ray of every fetus submitted for an autopsy is desirable. The views include: (1) An anteroposterior and lateral view of the entire fetus is preferable; (2) anterior, right-, and left-side views of the head; and (3) close-up views as and when required. A suspected diagnosis of skeletal dysplasia warrants additional radiographs **(Figs. 1A to C)**.

Photography

External and internal organ photographic documentation of the stillborn baby is of significance. The focus of the pictures must be to capture the abnormal with adequate anatomical reference points within the frame **(Figs. 2A and B)**.[1] If fetal fragments are received, then they are radiographed as well as photographed after spreading them in a single layer.[2]

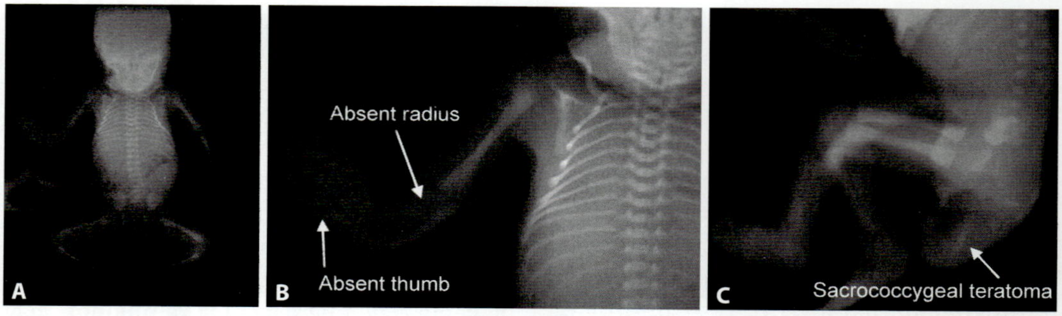

Figs. 1A to C: (A) Fetal X-ray; (B) Fetal X-ray with radial ray anomaly in a case of SALL-4 pathogenic variant Duane-radial ray/Okihiro syndrome; (C) Fetal X-ray in a case of sacrococcygeal teratoma.

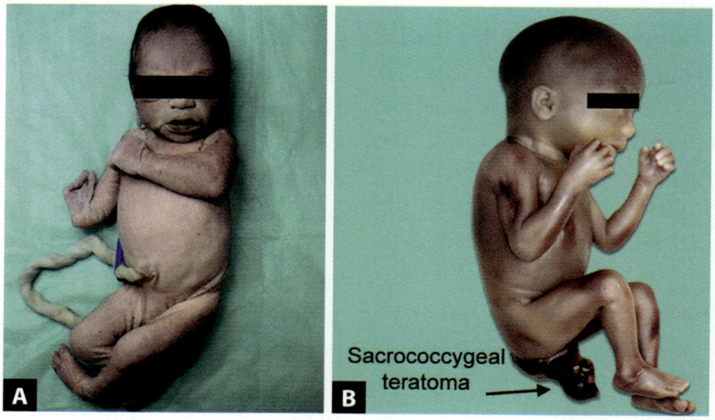

Figs. 2A and B: (A) External phenotype in a case of SALL-4 pathogenic variant Duane-radial ray/Okihiro syndrome; (B) External phenotype in a case sacrococcygeal teratoma.

Molecular and Cytogenetic Study

Samples for molecular and cytogenetic studies are usually taken from the skin over the chest at the main incision site or the axilla by using a sterile saline technique.[2] Alcohol usage is discouraged. For culture techniques, Achilles tendon, fascia, lungs, cartilage, and chorionic villous tissue are recommended. In skeletal dysplasia, suspected cases fibroblast culture is preferable. Bile, fresh frozen tissue, and fibroblast culture are used for suspected inborn errors of metabolism. In macerated fetuses, placental chorionic villous tissue may be sampled.[3] For electron, microscopic ultrastructural examination require tissue to be fixed in glutaraldehyde. Frozen nerve and skeletal muscle are sampled for hereditary neuromuscular disease evaluation.[2]

Perinatal Autopsy Instruments

For small fetuses, ophthalmic instruments work excellently.[1] The instruments **(Fig. 3)** and other requirements include: (1) Scalpel handles and blades; (2) a large knife; (3) small and medium-sized forceps with and without teeth; (4) stage scissors, metzenbaum scissors, and small scissors; (5) fine probes and hemostats of varying sizes; (6) measuring tape, rulers, and calipers; (7) large scale for large fetuses and electronic digital scale for internal organs; (8) dissecting board; (9) absorbent paper towels; (10) mounted

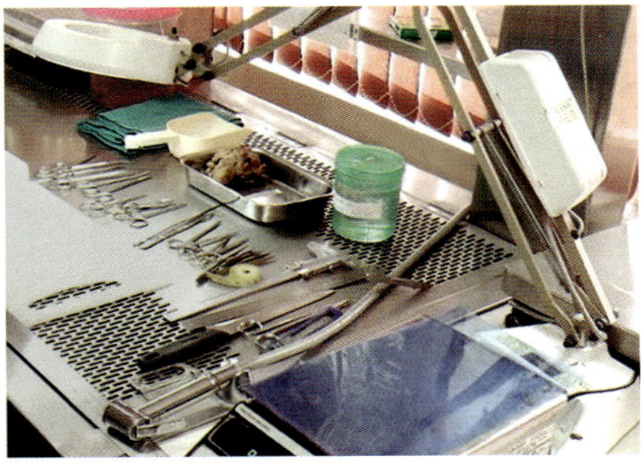

Fig. 3: Instruments used in fetal/perinatal autopsy.

magnifying glass; (11) sterile forceps and scissors for culture and karyotype; (12) sterile syringes and needles; (13) wedge-shaped autopsy block; and (14) charts providing standard normal weights and measurements for gestational age.

Initial Assessment

The initial step in the evaluation of a stillbirth requires assessment of fetal maceration.[3] Maceration is graded on a scale of 0–5 based on skin changes.[3] The maceration changes can be seen 4–6 hours after fetal death. The grades include: Grade 0—no maceration with the tissue appearing normal; grade I—skin desquamation involving ≤1% of total body surface and the umbilical cord shows brown-red discoloration; grade II—skin desquamation of face, abdomen, or back involving ≥1% and ≤5% of the total body surface. Internal serous fluid collection with tissue appearing red/pink or fresh with focal discoloration; grade III—skin desquamation involving >5% of body surface. Internal tissue appearing red/pink and mixed with brown; grade IV—complete brown discoloration of skin and internal tissue appearing brown/gray; and grade V—mummification and tissue appearing gray.[3,4]

External Examination

Systematic external examination of the stillborn is mandatory and is performed using standardized protocols.[5,6] It is best to proceed in a cephalocaudal direction, regardless of gestational age. Apart for maceration elucidated earlier, fetal dysmorphism, fetal growth, edema, dehydration, cyanosis, jaundice, meconium staining, and injuries related to delivery are some other features to be looked for.[1] The following measurements must be recorded: (1) Head circumference (HC); (2) chest circumference (CC); (3) abdominal circumference; (4) outer and inner canthal measurements (OC and IC); (5) interpupillary distance; (6) philtrum length; and (7) foot length.

Incision

A "Y"-shaped incision is employed. The arms of the "Y" incision begin from the tip of the shoulders, descend lateral and inferior to the nipples, and meet in the midline at the xiphoid process of the sternum. The incision is given by placing the fetus over a wedge-shaped autopsy block with hyperextended neck falling back over the wedge and shoulders and chest slightly raised.[1] The vertical stem of "Y" is extended caudally from the xiphoid, around the umbilicus to terminate at the symphysis pubis.[1]

In Situ Examination and Evisceration of Internal Organs

Traditionally, four fetal autopsy techniques have been described. These include: (1) Rokitansky method; (2) Virchow technique; (3) Letulle method; and (4) Gohn's technique.[1,5] The choice of technique is made by the dissector at the beginning of the autopsy with the sole intent of salvaging maximum information possible with minimal fetal mutilation.[1]

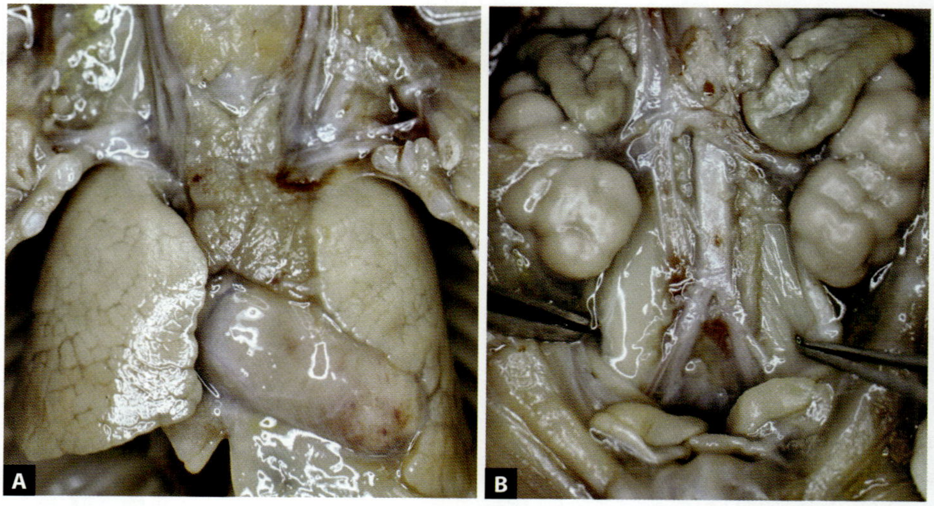

Figs. 4A and B: Four in-situ examination of internal organs: (A) Thoracic organs; (B) Renal organs.

The Rokitansky method is an in-situ examination of viscera **(Figs. 4A and B)**, in part combined with en bloc removal of internal organs. The Virchow technique involves that the internal organs are removed one by one and are dissected as removed. The Letulle method is an en masse removal of thoracic, cervical, abdominal, and pelvic organs with subsequent dissection into tissue organ blocks. The Gohn's technique is an en bloc removal of viscera into functionally related blocks and is deemed as a compromise between the Virchow and the Letulle methods. For step-by-step dissection methods, the reader is referred to specialized texts.[1,2,5,7]

Microscopic Examination

It is recommended that most if not all the internal organs are sampled for histologic examination. The tissue blocks must be submitted in a standardized order.[2,5,7] The sections are submitted for routine hematoxylin and eosin staining. Immunohistochemical stains are ordered as and when required and the most frequently used antibodies are for detecting viral infections such as cytomegalovirus, parvovirus B19, and herpes simplex.[2,7]

REFERENCES

1. Jaiman S. Performing a Perinatal Autopsy. J Fetal Med. 2015;2(3):101-11.
2. Pinar H, Koch MA, Hawkins H, Heim-Hall J, Abramowsky CR, Thorsten VR, et al. The stillbirth collaborative research network postmortem examination protocol. Am J Perinatol. 2012;29(3):187-202.
3. Genest DR, Singer DB. Estimating the time of death in stillborn fetuses: III. External fetal examination; a study of 86 stillborns. Obstet Gynecol. 1992;80(4):593-600.
4. Genest DR, Williams MA, Greene MF. Estimating the time of death in stillborn fetuses: I. Histologic evaluation of fetal organs; an autopsy study of 150 stillborns. Obstet Gynecol. 1992;80(4):575-84.
5. Gilbert-Barness E, Spicer DE, Steffensen TS (Eds). Handbook of Pediatric Autopsy Pathology, 2nd edition. Germany: Springer Nature; 2014. pp. 1-750.
6. Khong TY, Malcomson RDG (Eds). Keeling's Fetal and Neonatal Pathology, 5th edition. Switzerland AG: Springer International Publishing; 2015. p. 882.
7. Pinar H, Koch MA, Hawkins H, Heim-Hall J, Shehata B, Thorsten VR, et al. The Stillbirth Collaborative Research Network neuropathologic examination protocol. Am J Perinatol. 2011;28(10):793-802.

CHAPTER 17

Preconception and Prenatal Diagnostic Techniques Act

Reena Yadav

KEY POINTS

1. The Preconception and Prenatal Diagnostic Techniques (PC-PNDT) (Prohibition of Sex Selection) Act was enacted in 1994 and amended in 2002.
2. The objective of the Act is prohibition of sex selection, before and after conception.
3. The Act provides guidance regarding where, how, and when the prenatal diagnostic tests are to be done and by whom.
4. Prenatal diagnostic test according to the Act is that which is capable of sex selection; it includes ultrasonography (USG), analysis of amniotic fluid, chorionic villous sampling, fetal blood or any fluid, and fetoscopy.
5. Every center which wishes to do the prenatal diagnostic tests or wishes to procure an equipment capable of prenatal diagnosis (PND) needs to apply for registration by filling the A form in duplicate.
6. Only a person (medical geneticist, gynecologist, pediatrician, and registered medical practitioner) who possess prescribed qualification can do these tests only at registered place under the Act.
7. *Code of conduct:*
   - *Notice board:* Prohibiting seeking sex selection, certificate to be displayed, and copy of the Act to be kept near machine
   - Not to disclose sex in any manner
   - Maintenance of record forms—D, E, F, and G
   - Form for maintenance of permanent record (Form H)
   - Each center to send complete report of all preconception- and prenatal-related procedures/tests conducted by them every month by 5th day of following month to the concerned appropriate authority
   - Preserved for a period of 2 years from the date of completion of counseling, prenatal diagnostic procedure, or prenatal diagnostic test.

INTRODUCTION

The Prenatal Diagnostic Technique Act (regulation and prevention of misuse) came on the statute book as Prenatal Diagnostic Techniques Act, 1994 and Amendment Act 2002. The nomenclature of the Act amended and now it stands as "The Preconception and Prenatal Diagnostic Techniques (Prohibition of Sex Selection) Act, 1994."

The objectives of the Preconception and Prenatal Diagnostic Techniques Act are:

- Prohibition of sex selection, before and after conception
- Regulation of prenatal diagnostic techniques for the purpose of detecting genetic abnormalities or metabolic disorders or chromosomal abnormalities

or certain congenital malformation or sex-linked disorders
- Prevention of its misuse for sex determination leading to female feticide

The Act provides guidance regarding:
- Where should the prenatal diagnosis tests be done?
- Who should be doing the tests?
- When should the tests are to be done?
- What should be the code of conduct for the tests?
- What not to do?
- How the records are to be maintained?
- What happens if found guilty?

What comprises prenatal diagnostic test?
That which is capable of sex selection: Ultrasonography, analysis of amniotic fluid, chorionic villous sampling, fetal blood or any fluid, and fetoscopy.

Where should the test be done?
- *Genetic counseling center (GCC):* Institute, hospital, nursing home, or any place which provides genetic counseling to the patients
- *Genetic clinic (GC)/ultrasound clinic/imaging center:* Which is used for conducting prenatal diagnostic procedures
- Genetic *laboratory (GL):* Conducts analysis for prenatal diagnostic tests

Who can conduct prenatal diagnostic test?
- Only GCC, GL, and GC registered under the Act can conduct or associate with or help in conducting activities relating to prenatal diagnostic techniques.
- Only a person (medical geneticist, gynecologist, pediatrician, and registered medical practitioner) who possess prescribed qualification can do these tests only at registered place under the Act.
- *Medical geneticist:* A person who possesses a degree or diploma or certificate in medical genetic science in the field of *preconception techniques/*prenatal diagnostic techniques or has experience of not less than 2 years in such field after obtaining any one of the medical qualifications recognized under the Indian Medical Council Act, 1956 or postgraduate (PG) degree in biological sciences.

Who can run a GCC?
A gynecologist or a pediatrician having 6 months experience or 4 weeks training in genetic counseling or a medical geneticist.

Who can run a GL?
A medical geneticist or a laboratory technician having B.Sc. degree in biological sciences or degree or diploma in medical laboratory course with at least 1 year experience in conducting appropriate prenatal diagnostic techniques, tests, or procedures.

Who can run a GC/ultrasound clinic/imaging center?
A sonologist/imaging specialist, radiologist, or registered medical practitioner (RMP) having PG degree/diploma/6 months of training/1 year of experience in sonography or image scanning or a medical geneticist.

Who can do invasive procedures?
Any person being or employing—a gynecologist having experience of performing at least 20 procedures in chorionic villous aspirations per vagina/per abdomen, amniocentesis, cordocentesis/fetoscopy/fetal blood sampling (FBS)/tissue biopsy under supervision of experienced gynecologist in these fields (for invasive).

Sex selection on a woman or a man or both or on any tissue, embryo, conceptus, fluid, or gametes destined from either or both of them is prohibited.

The Act also states the prerequisites for equipment and space as follows:

- List of laboratory equipment
- List of additional facility for invasive center
- List for counseling center
- Sale of any ultrasound machine or imaging machine or scanner or any other equipment capable of detecting sex of fetus to any GCC, GL, and GC not registered under the Act is prohibited.

What is expected from GCC, GL, and GC according to the Act for conducting prenatal diagnostic test?

- Every center which wishes to do the prenatal diagnostic tests or wishes to procure an equipment capable of PND needs to register itself.
- Registration is always of the institute/ head of the institute or a person on his behalf.
- Registration application is submitted to appropriate authority (Form A)—in duplicate with an affidavit containing an undertaking to the effect that the center shall not conduct any test/procedure for selection of sex before/after conception or for detection of sex except for diseases specified in the Act.
- Qualified person proof, affidavit from the center, machine details, space available, and lease of the hospital building.
- Appropriate authority conducts inspection—the district approval committee recommends registration and subsequently, the approval is granted.

PROHIBITION OF COMMUNICATING THE SEX OF FETUS

- No person, including a relative or the husband of a woman, shall seek or encourage the conduct of any prenatal diagnostic technique on her except for the purpose specified in the clause.
- No person including the person conducting prenatal diagnostic procedures shall communicate to the pregnant woman concerned or her relatives or any other person the sex of the fetus by words, signs, or in any other manner.
- Advertisement
- No person, organization, GCC, GL, or GC, including clinic, laboratory, or center having ultrasound machine capable of undertaking determination of sex of fetus shall issue or cause to be issued any advertisement in any manner regarding facilities of prenatal determination of sex and preconception sex selection available at such center, laboratory, clinic, or any other place.

FORMS

- *Form D—counseling center:* Consists of details of patient and reasons for counseling. To be filled in all cases in which counseling is done
- *Form E—for GL:* Consists of details of patient and reasons for genetic tests. To be filled in all cases in which genetic test is done
- *Form F—for doing prenatal diagnostic procedure:* Consists of details of patient and reasons for counseling. To be filled in all cases in which prenatal diagnostic procedure is done on a pregnant woman. It has four parts—parts A, B, C, and D. Part C is to be filled only in cases where invasive procedure is done. Part D contains declaration by pregnant women that she does not want the sex of the baby to be revealed to her and also contains declaration by the doctor that the sex of the baby has not been detected by him or her.
- *Form G—for consent before invasive procedure:* Obtain a written consent (Form G)

in a language the person undergoing such procedure understands (Subrule 1A); it contains declaration by the doctor and declaration of the pregnant women. The concerned state government/union territory (UT) may issue translation of Form G in local languages.

- *Form H—record maintenance*: Register containing the information in serial order—patient's name and spouse's/father's name, age, address with contact number, number of children with sex, last menstrual period (LMP), indication, result of ultrasound (hard copy/digital record), referring doctor (with referral/self-referral slip preserved for cross-checking) and signature of radiologist and monthly closure, and date on which the patient first reported for genetic counseling/procedure/test as specified in Rule 9(1) of the Act should be maintained.

DETERMINATION OF SEX PROHIBITED

- Communication of the sex of her fetus by words, signs, or in any other manner to the concerned pregnant woman or her relations or any other person is prohibited.
- No GCC or GL or GC or any person can conduct or cause to be conducted prenatal diagnostic techniques, including USG for the purpose of determining the sex of the fetus.
- No person can cause or allow to be caused selection of sex before or after conception.
- No GL shall accept for analysis or test any sample unless referred to it by GC.
- Every prenatal diagnostic procedure shall invariably immediately be preceded by locating the fetus and placenta by USG and procedure to be done under direct USG monitoring so as to prevent damage to the fetus and placenta.

WHO REGULATES THE RECOMMENDATIONS?

- Central government constitutes a central supervisory board.
- Government of each state constitutes a state supervisory board.

CONSTITUTION OF CENTRAL ADVISORY BOARD

- Under the Act, the board is constituted by central government to exercise the powers and to perform the functions conferred on the board.
- The board consists of:
  - Chairman—minister of Ministry of Health and Family Welfare (MOHFW) Ex-Officio
  - Vice chairperson—secretary to Government of India, MOHFW Ex-Officio
  - Three members appointed by central government to represent ministries of women and child development, department of legal affairs/ministry of law and justice, and Indian system of medicine and homeopathy
  - Directorate General Health Services (DGHS) of central government
  - Ten members appointed by central government, two each from amongst:
    - Eminent medical geneticists
    - Eminent gynecologists and obstetrician
    - Eminent pediatrician
    - Eminent social scientist
    - Representative of women welfare organization
  - Three women members of parliament

- Four members to be appointed by the central government by rotation to represent the states and union territories
- Member secretary—an officer, not below the rank of Joint Secretary or equivalent of central government, in charge of family welfare

Functions of the Board

- To advise the central government on the policy matters relating to use of prenatal diagnostic techniques and sex selection techniques against their misuse
- To review and monitor implementation of the Act and Rules made there under and recommend to central government changes in the said Act and Rules
- To create public awareness against the practice of preconception sex selection and prenatal determination of sex of fetus leading to female feticide
- To lay down code of conduct to be observed by persons working at GCC, GL, and GC
- To oversee the performance of various bodies constituted under the Act and taken appropriate steps to ensure its proper and effective implementation
- Any other functions as may be prescribed under the Act

APPROPRIATE AUTHORITY AND ADVISORY COMMITTEE

- Central Government shall appoint by notification in official gazette one or more appropriate authority for each union territory.
- Similarly, state government shall appoint by notification in official gazette one or more appropriate authority for state for the purpose of this Act.
- Appropriate authority consisting of following members:
  - An officer of or above the rank of joint director of health and family welfare—chairperson
  - An eminent woman representing women's organization
  - An officer of law department of the state or union territory concerned

Functions of Appropriate Authority

- To grant, suspend, or cancel registration of a GCC, GL, or GC
- To enforce standard prescribed for the GCC, GL, and CG
- To investigate complaints of breach of the provisions of the Act or the Rules made and take immediate action
- To seek and consider the advice of advisory committee on application for registration and on complaints for suspension or cancellation of registration
- To take appropriate legal action against the use of any sex selection techniques by any person at any place brought to its notice and also to initiate independent investigation in such matters
- To create public awareness against the practice of sex selection or prenatal determination of sex
- To supervise the implementation of the provisions of the Act and Rules
- To recommend to the board and state boards modification required in the Rules in accordance with changes in technology or social conditions
- To take action on the recommendation of advisory committee made after investigation of complaint for suspension or cancellation registration

REGISTRATION OF GENETIC COUNSELING CENTERS, GENETIC LABORATORIES, AND GENETIC CLINIC

- Every application for registration in duplicate shall be made to the appropriate authority in such form (*Form A*) and in such manner and shall be accompanied by such fees (INR 25,000/-) for GCC/GL/GC, ultrasound clinic, or imaging center and INR 35,000/- for an institute, hospital, nursing home, or any place providing such services as may be prescribed.
- An undertaking to the effect that genetic center/laboratory/clinic/ultrasound clinic/imaging center as the case may be, shall not conduct any test or procedure for selection of sex before or after conception except for diseases specified under the Act and shall display prominently a notice that they do not conduct any technique, test, procedure, etc. for detection of sex before or after conception.
- No government institute which provides health and medical services shall be required to pay fee for registration and renewal of registration.
- No GCC/laboratory/clinic shall be registered under the Act unless appropriate authority is satisfied that such center/laboratory/clinic is in a position to provide such facilities and maintain such equipment and standard as may be prescribed.
- No GCC/laboratory/clinic including any of them having ultrasound or imaging machine or scanner or any other technology capable of undertaking the determination of sex of fetus and sex selection can be opened unless it is duly registered under the Act.

Certificate of Registration

- Appropriate authority shall, after holding an inquiry and after satisfying itself that applicant has complied with all the requirements of the Act and Rules made there under and having regard to the advice of Advisory committee in this behalf, grant a certificate of registration in duplicate in the prescribed form (*Form B*) to the GCC/laboratory/clinic/ultrasound clinic or imaging center as the case may be.
- Provided that appropriate authority may grant a certificate of registration to a GL or a GC to conduct one or more specified prenatal diagnostic tests or procedures depending upon the availability of place, equipment, qualified employees, and standard maintained by such laboratory or clinic.
- Every certificate of registration shall be renewed in such manner (*Form A*) and after such period (5 years), within 30 days of expiry of the certificate of registration and on payment of such fees (half of the fees for first registration) as may be prescribed.
- The certificate of registration shall be displayed by the registered GCC/laboratory/clinic, ultrasound clinic or imaging center in a conspicuous place at its place of business.
- If after enquiry and after giving an opportunity of being heard to the applicant and having regard to the advice of advisory committee, the appropriate authority is satisfied that applicant has not complied with the requirements of the Act and these Rules, it shall for the reasons to be recorded in writing, reject the application for registration and communicate such rejection to the applicant as specified in *Form C*.

- Grant of certificate of registration or rejection of application for registration shall be communicated to the applicant in Form B or Form C, as the case may be, within a period of 90 days after date of receipt of application for registration.
- The certificate of registration is nontransferable. In case of change of ownership, the new owner of such place shall apply afresh for grant of certificate and both copies of previous certificate shall be surrendered to the appropriate authority.

Cancellation and Suspension of Registration

- The appropriate authority may, on complaint, issue a notice to the GCC/laboratory/clinic to show cause why its registration should not be suspended or cancelled for the reasons mentioned in the notice.
- If after giving reasonable opportunity of being heard to the GCC/GL/GC and having regard to the advice of advisory committee, the appropriate authority is satisfied that there is breach of the provisions of this Act or the Rules, it may suspend its registration for such period as it may think fit or cancel the registration as the case may be.
- Appropriate authority has the power to suspend or cancel registration even without issuing a show cause notice if it is of opinion that it is necessary or expedient so as to do in the public interest.

Appeal

The GCC/GL/GC may within 30 days from date of receipt of the order of suspension or cancellation of registration passed by the appropriate authority prefer an appeal against such order to central government where the appeal is against the order of central appropriate authority or the state government where the appeal is against the state appropriate authority.

OFFENCES AND PENALTIES—PROHIBITION OF ADVERTISEMENT RELATING TO PC-PNDT DETERMINATION OF SEX AND PUNISHMENT OF CONTRAVENTION

- No person organization, GCC/GL/GC, including clinic having USG machine, imaging machine or scanner, or any other technology capable of sex determination of fetus or sex selection shall advertise in any form (notice, circular, label, wrapper, any document including internet/media/electronic or print) regarding facilities of prenatal determination of sex or sex selection before conception available at such center.
- Any person who contravenes the provisions shall be punishable with imprisonment for a term which may extend to 3 years and with fine which may extend to INR 10,000 and on any subsequent conviction, with imprisonment which may extend to 5 years and fine which may extend to INR 50,000.
- The name of the registered medical practitioner shall be reported by appropriate authority to the State Medical (SM) council concerned for taking necessary action including suspension of the registration if the charges are framed by the court and till the case is disposed of and on conviction for removal of his name from the register of medical council for a period of 5 years for the first offence and permanently for subsequent offence.

- Any person who seeks for sex selection or for conducting prenatal diagnostic technique on any pregnant person for the purpose other than those specified under the Act shall be punishable with imprisonment for a term which may extend to 3 years and with fine which may extend to INR 50,000 for first offence and for any subsequent offence with imprisonment up to 5 years and fine up to INR 100,000. This will not be applicable to woman who was compelled to undergo such diagnostic techniques.
- Offences to be cognizable, nonbailable, and noncompoundable

Cognizance of Offence

- No court shall take cognizance of an offence under the Act except on a complaint made by:
    - The appropriate authority or any officer authorized in the behalf by central government or state government as the case may be
    - A person has been given notice of not less than 15 days in the manner prescribed to the appropriate authority of alleged offence and his intention to make a complaint to the court
- No court other than that of Metropolitan Magistrate or a Judicial Magistrate of the first class shall try any offence punishable under the Act.

MAINTENANCE OF RECORDS

- Every GCC/GL/GC/ultrasound clinic and imaging center shall maintain a register showing serial order, name, and addresses of the men or women given genetic counseling, subjected to prenatal diagnostic procedures/tests, and the name of their spouse and date on which they first reported for such counseling, procedure, or test.
- For GCC in Form D, for GL in Form E, and for GC including a mobile GC in Form F
- The appropriate authority shall maintain a permanent record of applications for grant or renewal of certificate of registration as specified in Form H.
- Letters of intimation of every change of employee, place, address, and equipment installed shall also be preserved as permanent record.
- All records, charts, forms, reports, consent forms, and all the documents are required to be maintained under this Act and the Rules shall be preserved for a period of 2 years. But if criminal or other proceedings are instituted against any center, the records and all other documents of such center shall be preserved till the final disposal of such proceedings and shall be made available for inspection of appropriate authority.
- In case the center maintains records on computer or other electronic equipment, a printed copy of the record shall be taken and preserved after authentication by a person responsible for such record.
- Appropriate authority has the power to search and seize and seal records if such authority has reason to believe that it may furnish evidence of the commission of offence punishable under the Act.

FACILITIES FOR INSPECTION

- All such centers shall ensure all reasonable facilities for inspection of the place, equipment, and records to the appropriate authority or any other person authorized by the appropriate authority in this behalf for registration of such institutions under the Act or for detection of misuse of such facilities or advertisement for selection of sex before or after conception or for detection/disclosure of sex of fetus or for violation of the provisions of Act in any other manner.

- The appropriate authority or the officer authorized by it may seal and seize USG machine or any other equipment used by any organization if organization has not got itself registered under the Act and further action as per provisions of the Act.

PROCEDURE FOR SEARCH AND SEIZURE

- The appropriate authority or any officer authorized in this behalf may enter and search at all reasonable time any center/ organization in the presence of two or more independent witnesses for the purpose of search and examination of any record, register, document, book, pamphlet, advertisement, or any other material object found therein seal and seize the same if there is reason to believe that it may furnish evidence of commission of an offence punishable under the Act.
- A list of such documents found in the center/organization seized shall be prepared in duplicate at the place of effecting the seizure. Both copies of such list shall be signed on each page by appropriate authority or by an officer authorized in this behalf and by the witnesses to the seizure.
- One copy of the list shall be handed over under acknowledgment to the person from whose custody records/ documents have been seized; if no person acknowledges, then list may be delivered under acknowledgment to the owner/ manager by registered post.

Intimation in changes in employee, place, or equipment—shall be intimated to the appropriate authority at least 30 days in advance to the expected date of such change and seek reissue of certificate of registration with the changes duly incorporated.

PROTECTION OF ACTION TAKEN IN GOOD FAITH

No legal proceedings shall lie against central or state government or the appropriate authority or any officer authorized by them for anything which is done in good faith.

PUBLIC INFORMATION

- Every GCC/clinic/laboratory/ultrasound clinic and imaging center shall prominently display on its premises a notice in English and in the local language for information of the public, to the effect that disclosure of the sex of the fetus is prohibited under the law.
- One copy each of the Act and these Rules shall be available on the premises of every center and shall be available to clientele on demand for perusal.
- The appropriate authority may publish list of registered centers periodically and other information in their possession for information of the public and for use by the experts in the field.

CODE OF CONDUCT TO BE OBSERVED BY PERSONS WORKING AT GENETIC COUNSELING CENTERS/ LABORATORIES/CLINIC/ ULTRASOUND CLINIC/ IMAGING CENTER

- Not conduct or associate with or help in carrying out detection or disclosure of sex of the fetus in any manner
- Not employ any person not having not possessing qualification necessary

for carrying out prenatal diagnostic technique/procedures and tests, including USG
- Ensure that no provision of the Act and these Rules are violated in any manner
- Help law-enforcing agencies in bringing to book the violators of the provisions of the Act and these Rules
- Display his/her name prominently on the dress worn
- Write his/her name in full under his/her signature

POWER TO MAKE RULES

- The central government may make rules for carrying out the provisions of this Act regarding minimum qualification of persons employed at a registered center, manner in which records to be kept, the form of consent, procedure to be followed by members of central supervisory board in discharge of their functions, allowance of members, code of conduct to be observed by genetic centers, the manner in which reports shall be furnished by state/union territory supervisory board to central government, empowering the appropriate authority in any other matter, the term and conditions of appointment of persons to advisory committee and procedure to be followed by such committee, the form and manner in which application shall be made for registration and fee payable, the facility provided, equipment, and other standard to be maintained by GCC/GL/GC, the form in which certificate shall be issued, period after which renewal is required, the manner in which appeal is preferred, the period up to which record shall be preserved, and the manner in which documents to be seized and list prepared.
- Every rule and every regulation made under the Act shall be laid as soon as it is formulated before each house of parliament.

OFFENCES AND PENALTIES

- Any offence under this law is cognizable, nonbailable, and noncompoundable.
- Appropriate authority can inspect anytime and seize the machine and records in case of omission of rules.
- *Punishment for the offences by persons*:
    - *First offence:* 3 years imprisonment and fine of INR 10,000/-
    - *Subsequent offences:* 5 years imprisonment and fine up to INR 50,000/-
- *Suspension by SM council and removal of name from register of Medical Council of India (MCI)*:
    - *First offence:* For 5 years
    - *Subsequent offence:* Permanently
- *Patient or attendant*: 3 months imprisonment and INR 1,000/- or both

SUGGESTED READING

1. The Pre-conception and Pre-natal Diagnostic techniques (Prohibition of Sex Selection) Act 1994 (As amended by the J&K reorganisation Act 2019).
2. The Pre-conception and Pre-natal Diagnostic techniques (Prohibition of Sex Selection) Rules 1996.
3. The Pre-conception and Pre-natal Diagnostic techniques (Prohibition of Sex Selection) (Six months training) Rules 2014.

Quiz 2

Bijoya Mukherjee, Akshatha Prabhu

1. Expression of certain genes varies based on the sex of the parent from whom they were inherited. This concept is known as:
   a. Uniparental disomy
   b. Mitochondrial inheritance
   c. Imprinting
   d. Triple repeat disorders
2. What would be the risk of recurrence for cystic fibrosis if one parent is affected and the other is a carrier?
   a. 100% b. 50%
   c. 25% d. 12.5%
3. Fragile X syndrome follows rules of:
   a. Mendelian inheritance
   b. Nonmendelian inheritance
   c. Imprinting
   d. Mitochondrial inheritance
4. Once the risk of recurrence has been arrived at which of the following should not be offered as a part of reproductive options available to the couple:
   a. Prenatal diagnosis through chorionic villus sampling or amniocentesis
   b. IVF with preimplantation genetic testing (PGT)
   c. IVF with donor oocyte or sperm
   d. Surrogacy
5. Which of the following are inherited in an autosomal dominant fashion?
   a. Achondroplasia
   b. Spinal muscular atrophy
   c. Osteogenesis imperfecta
   d. Marfan syndrome
6. First-trimester quadruple test includes:
   a. BhCG, PAPP-A, PlGF, alpha-fetoprotein (AFP)
   b. BhCG, PlGF, inhibin-A (InhA), AFP
   c. BhCG, PAPP-A, InhA, AFP
   d. PlGF, PAPP-A, InhA, AFP
7. Which of the following is true?
   a. Noninvasive prenatal testing (NIPT) (cell-free fetal DNA) is the only screening test for Down syndrome
   b. NIPT is the test of choice for increased NT
   c. Small deletions and duplications can be picked up by karyotype
   d. Quadruple test has the highest sensitivity among the screening tests for Down syndrome
8. The additional yield of chromosomal microarray over karyotype analysis is:
   a. 6–10% b. 10–15%
   c. 15–20% d. >20%
9. Multiplex ligation-dependent probe amplification (MLPA) study is best suited for:
   a. Angelman syndrome
   b. Prader–Willi syndrome
   c. Spinomuscular atrophy
   d. All of the above
10. The most accurate and informative genetic testing for monogenic disorders is:
    a. Proband whole-exome sequencing
    b. Trio whole-exome sequencing
    c. Chromosomal microarray
    d. Karyotype analysis

11. Most common congenital anomaly detected prenatally:
    a. Cardiovascular system (CVS)
    b. Central nervous system (CNS)
    c. Gastrointestinal tract (GIT)
    d. Limb malformations
12. Percentage of prenatal detection of open neural tube defect (NTD) is:
    a. 100% b. >90%
    c. 80% d. 75%
13. Which of the following is true?
    a. Holoprosencephaly can be detected in the first trimester
    b. Gastroschisis cannot be picked up in the first trimester
    c. Imperforate anus has a good prenatal detection rate
    d. Fetal structural abnormalities are seen in 7% of all pregnancies
14. Coarctation of aorta is usually detected on ultrasound in:
    a. First trimester
    b. Second trimester
    c. Third trimester
    d. Postnatally
15. First-trimester screening [Fetal Medicine Foundation (FMF)] includes:
    a. Down syndrome screening
    b. Down syndrome screening + early structural anomalies survey
    c. Screening for T21, T18, 13 + early structural anomalies survey
    d. None of the above
16. Which of the following is false?
    a. Rubella vaccination should be given to nonimmune nonpregnant women of childbearing age
    b. Toxoplasma vaccination is available.
    c. Fetal cytomegalovirus (CMV) infection causes brain damage
    d. Chickenpox in pregnancy can affect 0.8–2% of the fetuses
17. Periventricular calcifications and subependymal cysts are ultrasound signs suggestive of:
    a. Toxoplasma
    b. CMV
    c. Rubella
    d. Both a and b
18. The leading nongenetic cause of sensorineural hearing loss is:
    a. Rubella
    b. CMV
    c. Herpes
    d. Toxoplasma
19. Maternal serology testing—rubella immunoglobulin (IgG) positive, IgM positive, avidity testing high—suggestive of:
    a. Infection more than 3 months ago
    b. Secondary infection
    c. Infection within 3 months
    d. Either a or b
20. The risk of fetal infection is highest in case of maternal infection with varicella zoster at:
    a. <13 weeks b. 13–20 weeks
    c. 24–36 weeks d. >37 weeks
21. Placentomegaly in second trimester is defined as placental thickness more than:
    a. 5 cm b. 4 cm
    c. 10 cm d. 6 cm
22. The most common etiology of nonimmune hydrops is:
    a. GIT abnormalities
    b. CVS anomalies
    c. Infections
    d. Genetic causes
23. Chylothorax/lymphatic is mainly associated with:
    a. Edward's syndrome
    b. Noonan syndrome
    c. Patau's syndrome
    d. Down syndrome

24. Which fetal enzyme is raised in nonimmune hydrops (NIH) with bowel perforation?
    a. Alkaline phosphatase (ALP)
    b. Gamma-glutamyl transpeptidase (GGT)
    c. Serum glutamyl oxalate transaminase (SGOT)
    d. Serum glutamyl pyruvate transaminase (SGPT)
25. Idiopathic NIH is present in:
    a. 60% cases b. 40% cases
    c. 30% cases d. 50% cases
26. NT between >99th centile at 12 weeks of gestation is an indication for:
    a. NIPT
    b. Dual marker
    c. CVS
    d. Expectant management
27. Early CVS (<10 weeks) is not indicated due to:
    a. Orofacial defects
    b. Limb reduction defects
    c. Cardiovascular defects
    d. High rate of miscarriage
28. Down syndrome screening in presence of one vanishing twin and one live twin in dichorionic diamniotic (DCDA) twin pregnancy on ultrasound is by:
    a. Ultrasound markers for Down syndrome
    b. Ultrasound markers for Down syndrome + maternal biochemistry
    c. NIPT
    d. None of the above
29. Turnaround time (TAT) for CMA is:
    a. 21 days
    b. 10–12 days
    c. 5–7 days
    d. >4 weeks
30. Possibility of heterokaryotypia in monochorionic diamniotic (MCDA) twin pregnancy necessitates genetic testing from:
    a. Amniotic fluid of one sac
    b. Amniotic fluid of two sacs
    c. Placenta
    d. None of the above

ANSWERS

1. c	2. b	3. b	4. d	5. a, c, d
6. a	7. a	8. a	9. d	10. b
11. a	12. b	13. a	14. c	15. c
16. b	17. d	18. b	19. d	20. b
21. a	22. b	23. b	24. b	25. b
26. c	27. b	28. a	29. b	30. b

Index

Page numbers followed by *b* refer to box, *f* refer to figure, *fc* refer to flowchart, and *t* refer to table.

A

B

C

I

J

K

L

M

Q

R

U

V

W

X

Y

Z